Ayurveda

Essential Ayurvedic Principles and Practices to Balance and Heal Naturally

(Unleashing the Power of the Ayurvedic Diet Yoga Meditation for Healing)

Gary Barrow

I0136083

Published By **Jackson Denver**

Gary Barrow

Ayurveda: Essential Ayurvedic Principles and Practices to Balance and Heal Naturally (Unleashing the Power of the Ayurvedic Diet Yoga Meditation for Healing)

ISBN   978-1-7388580-6-4

No part of this guidebook shall be reproduced in any form without permission in writing from the publisher except in the case of brief quotations embodied in critical articles or reviews.

Legal & Disclaimer

The information contained in this book is not designed to replace or take the place of any form of medicine or professional medical advice. The information in this book has been provided for educational & entertainment purposes only.

The information contained in this book has been compiled from sources deemed reliable, and it is accurate to the best of the Author's knowledge; however, the Author cannot guarantee its accuracy and validity and cannot be held liable for any errors or omissions. Changes are periodically made to this book. You must consult your doctor or get professional medical advice before using any of the suggested remedies, techniques, or information in this book.

Table Of Contents

Chapter 1: Basic Principles of Ayurvedic Medicine

Now that we've got were given a extra clean facts of what our lifestyles is comprised of, let's examine the number one standards of Ayurveda and the way they affect us.

What is the Philosophy and Principles of Ayurvedic Medicine?

According to Ayurveda, all of us is taken into consideration as a completely precise character who's made from 5 number one factors along with air, space, water, fireplace and earth. We derive those factors from the person. The weather and the meals we consume are the examples of the presence of those elements in the nature. When any of these elements are in an imbalance within the environment, they, in turn, have an negative have an impact on on us. Besides those five easy elements, there are advantageous different factors that seem to have an capability to create and help various physiological competencies in our frame.

The 3 Doshas in Ayurveda

The five number one factors integrate to shape the three doshas or bio-energies - vata, pitta and kapha – that form the bottom for the treatment in Ayurveda. Ayurveda believes that the functioning of all of the nature's creations together with people, plant life and animals can be understood because the interactions of these 3 number one doshas or electricity complexes. The 3 energies collectively represent the cellular or dynamic, non-fabric, transformative, active, clever, structural and physical factors of nature.

Firstly, air and area integrate to form what's known as the Vata dosha in Ayurveda. The phrase Vata stems from the Sanskrit word 'Vayu', because of this that 'something that actions'. It is considered the most influential dosha because of the truth it is the transferring stress within the again of kapha and pitta. It controls the precept of motion and is seen as a strain, which directs the capabilities which includes circulation, nerve impulses, breathing and elimination. Vata electricity is stated to be maximum vital in those who are modern, lively and function a flare for innovation. A vata-dominant man or woman is alert, short and stressed. She or he can also communicate, walk and assume short; however, might also additionally show the signs and symptoms of nervousness, fear and anxiety. When out-of-stability, this strength can motive joint pains, dry pores and pores and pores and skin, constipation and tension.

The one-of-a-kind 2 elements - Fire and water - integrate to shape the Pitta dosha, which courses the approach of metabolism or transformation. The term Pitta originates from the Sanskrit word 'Pinj', because of this 'to polish'. This dosha is idea to feature luster to the eyes, hair and the pores and pores and skin. The conversion of meals into vitamins just so the frame can use it as an electricity deliver is an instance of a pitta characteristic. Pitta is also responsible for the metabolism within the tissue structures and organs. Pitta is likewise concept to control the endocrinal features. People with pitta electricity are clever, aggressive achievers, fiery in temperament and speedy-paced. Pitta-dominant people additionally revel in a hearty urge for food and an efficient metabolism. But, whilst this power is out of balance, it may result in infection, ulcers, anger, heartburn, digestive issues and arthritis.

Finally, it's far the earth and water factors that combine to form the Kapha dosha. Kapha is a time period derived from the Sanskrit phrase 'Shlish', because of this 'some thing that holds subjects together'. It governs immunity and the strategies of self-repair and recuperation. This dosha is accountable for the boom of structures unit by using the usage of unit. Kapha also gives protection to the body tissues. Cerebrospinal fluid that protects the mind and the spinal column and the mucosal lining of the belly that protects the gastric tissues are the varieties of Kapha within the body. It offers physical staying power and psychological strength on the same time as selling human emotions like love, forgiveness, compassion, know-how, empathy, loyalty and persistence. Kapha-dominant human beings are tenacious but calm, robust but loving and are blessed with smart tolerance. But, even as this strength is out of balance, it can result in weight issues, diabetes, lack of confidence, sinus troubles and gallbladder illnesses.

Our frame and thoughts are in balance even as the ones types of 3 doshas are within the proper proportions. Optimal health is completed while those doshas are in concord with the soul, senses and thoughts.

The body of all people is created from a completely unique share of Vata, Pitta and Kapha. This is the reason for why Ayurveda sees each affected person as a unique man or woman with a very precise mixture, which debts for our range. Hence, it designs a completely precise remedy protocol to in particular cope with a person's fitness challenges. When any of those doshas will become excessive, Ayurveda indicates specific nutritional suggestions and life-style to assist the patient in reducing the dosha that has gathered. Ayurveda can also additionally endorse tremendous natural medicinal tablets to hasten the balancing way.

An imbalance can also get up even as one or extra of those factors are altered qualitatively. All types of situations that people enjoy including a belief, the weather, an emotion, food or way of lifestyles could have an impact at the physiological abilities of the frame.

What is 'Panchakarma'?

'Panchakarma' is the remedy of Purification. Panchakarma is typically recommended when there can be an accumulation of volatile pollution within the body. It is a cleansing manner that lets in to dispose of those undesirable pollution. It is a five-fold purification treatment, which paperwork the classical method of treatment in ayurveda. These specialised methods include of the following:

- Vaman (Therapeutic vomiting)

- Virechan (Purgation)

- Basti (Enema)

- Nasya (Elimination of pollutants through the nose)

- Rakta moksha (Bloodletting or detoxification of the blood)

What is Prakruti?

We already learnt that, in a human frame, the three doshas interact in a compensatory and harmonious way to govern and preserve life. Their relative expression in a person implies a very unique percentage of these bio-energies based totally on his or her particular DNA shape determined at concept. This is referred to as Prakruti or the frame typing of someone.

Prakruti is the specific constitution that people are born with. It can be seemed as a very specific aggregate of intellectual and bodily characteristics that determine the manner the person features. Throughout existence, the underlying Prakruti of an character remains the equal. However, it's far continuously stimulated via numerous inner and out of doors factors like seasonal changes, day and night time time time, way of life selections and weight loss plan. Ayurveda places emphasis at the prevention of illnesses, thru way of keeping fitness via seasonal and life-style regimens, which assist create stability.

The implication of Prakruti permits explain why patients react in a superb manner to the identical subjects. The clinical utility of that is positive human beings have a natural sensitivity to splendid drugs, which ends up in them developing tremendous facet outcomes, at the equal time as others react to the identical drug treatments in a remarkable way leading to finish treatment of the infection.

Chapter 2: Diagnostic techniques in Ayurveda

Diagnosis is a very critical difficulty of every tool of medication. Ayurveda, too, places masses of emphasis on diagnosing the contamination and the basis cause of the identical. Ayurveda, except relieving the physical signs and symptoms and signs of the contamination, moreover treats the person as an entire. Unless a right evaluation of the scenario is finished, it is tough to begin the right treatment and to remedy the infection certainly.

The idea of causative elements in Ayurveda

In Ayurveda, the analysis of a ailment is person to each patient. The root motive of any contamination may be internal or out of doors and regularly varies among specific human beings. All the causative elements of the sickness, directly or now not at once, create an imbalance inside the 3 doshas i.E. Vata, Pitta and Kapha, due to which the man or woman starts offevolved offevolved experiencing the unpleasant signs and symptoms and symptoms. The elements

9

affecting the health may be faulty eating regimen, way of life or each day sports activities. To provide long lasting remedy, this root purpose needs to be eliminated.

Diagnostic equipment in Ayurveda

Ayurveda makes use of five kinds of tools for comparing a scenario. These 5 techniques are known as Pancha Nidana; 'Pancha' because of this '5' and 'Nidana' because of this 'diagnostic techniques'. These 5 strategies are nidana (the purpose), purva rupa (preliminary signs and symptoms), rupa (symptoms), upashaya (exploratory strategies) and samprapti (illness development). Now allow's take a deeper observe the five diagnostic strategies in Ayurveda.

Nidana – The Causative thing

Nidana is the issue that causes the illness. Several elements like food regimen, way of existence, accidents or environmental variations that can disturb the doshas fall on this elegance. Indentifying the correct additives or unique sports sports that could get worse a dosha can assist us avoid the ones triggering factors and thereby prevent the superiority or relapse of the illness. Ayurveda offers a number of importance to 'Nidana parivarjana' which means that 'averting the reason'. It is taken into consideration the number one line of treatment for maximum of the ailments.

Purvarupa – The preliminary signs and symptoms

Purva rupa approach the preliminary signs and symptoms and signs and symptoms of a disorder. These signs begin performing masses before the actual onset of the contamination and often function a caution sign that the ailment can also take place soon. Most illnesses have particular set of preliminary signs and symptoms and signs and symptoms. For instance, in sufferers with epilepsy, the signs and symptoms and symptoms and signs and symptoms encompass feeling of any abnormal taste or scent, dimness of imaginative and prescient and a throbbing sensation anywhere within the body.

Rupa – The Symptoms

Rupa shows the real manifestation of the contamination. The disorder turns into extra said even as the plain and in reality defined symptoms and signs and symptoms begin appearing. The rupa is considered a complicated form of the purva rupa (caution symptoms and signs and symptoms and signs and symptoms). The big variety and the severity of the signs and signs and symptoms provide the medical medical doctor a clue for predicting the physical impact of the contamination, the opportunity of remedy (analysis) and the duration of time desired for complete restoration to take region.

Upashaya – The Exploratory Treatment

Certain illnesses have comparable reasons, caution signs and symptoms and symptoms and signs and symptoms and symptoms. For instance, fever may be a sign of malaria, dengue, typhoid or pneumonia. In historical times, at the same time as the contemporary-day diagnostic techniques were now not to be had, the analysis changed into aided through upashaya. It includes the detection and removal of sicknesses via adjustments in diet, physical treatment plans and herbal treatments, which help to confirm the prognosis.

For example, inside the case of fever, the medical doctor regularly begins offevolved the treatment with Quinine to look if the symptoms and symptoms are relieved. If that is executed, it confirms that the affected character had malaria. If affected person does no longer reply to Quinine, malaria can be ruled out. Similarly, dietary adjustments additionally can be encouraged to verify an opinion approximately a suspected evaluation.

Samprapti - Development of a illness

The word Samprapti comes from 'Samyak', this means that 'proper' and 'Prapti', because of this that 'to get'. Samprapti method to have the proper facts of the collection of disorder manifestation. It offers entire records of the development of the illness, beginning from the causative detail and the doshas involved. It consists of all the changes within the body taking place from the time of exposure to the motive to the real onset of the ailment and its manifestations.

Benefits of Pancha Nidana

Pancha Nidana aids in identifying the man or woman of the contamination, its location and an powerful mode of treatment. It additionally helps inside the prevention of the sickness by means of using providing an know-how of the causative aspect (nidana). Avoiding exposure to the causative factors and taking the proper precautions can assist human beings save you the infection in destiny.

Similarly, having understanding about the preliminary symptoms and symptoms of a ailment (purva rupa and rupa), can help a scientific health practitioner advise steps to fight the disease at an preliminary degree, before it flares up and motives complications.

Similarly, the sickness pathway (samprapti) and exploratory treatments (upashaya) allow an in-intensity information of unique additives of an contamination and allow a health practitioner to refine the remedy approach so you can make certain a eternal remedy. Therefore, the information of Pancha Nidana is especially valuable inside the analysis of ailments in particular the ones having comparable abilities.

Here are a few distinctive techniques of assessment used in Ayurveda for detecting the cause:

Pulse Diagnosis

Pulse analysis is a exceedingly effective tool utilized by ayurvedic practitioners for diagnosing the contamination. For an ayurvedic practitioner, taking the heart beat is more than certainly counting the beats. The health and functioning of the entire thoughts-frame device may be determined from the coronary coronary heart beat. It moreover allows in figuring out the imbalance of the doshas, the health of the numerous organs and the caution signs of capability fitness issues that could crop up in future.

The affected individual ought to be as near as feasible to his norm to get an correct pulse. The function of the index finger shows the

Vata dosha. If the vata is strong inside the man or woman, the index finger will experience a strong push of the coronary heart beat. A sturdy pulse in competition to the center finger shows the Pitta dosha. When the heart beat feels stronger beneath the ring finger, it's far the sign of Kapha charter.

Eye Diagnosis

Vata eyes seem small with dry, scanty lashes and drooping eyelids. The cornea appears muddy and the iris is black or gray-brown. Pitta eyes are moderate in length and seem sharp and lustrous. The lashes are oily and scanty. Kapha eyes are big and delightful with prolonged and thick lashes.

Tongue Diagnosis

A whitish tongue shows an imbalance in Kapha even as a yellowish-inexperienced or red tongue suggests a Pitta imbalance. A vata imbalance is manifested by means of using a brown or black discoloration on the tongue.

Facial Diagnosis

Ayurveda believes that the face is a replicate of the mind. Mental similarly to physical problems are manifested on the face in the shape of discoloration, wrinkles and lines. For example, immoderate horizontal wrinkling on the forehead can be a sign of deep-seated anxieties or issues. Full and fluffy decrease eyelids may additionally detail within the course of impaired kidneys.

The nostril may be used for figuring out the dosha of someone. People with dominant Vata have crooked nostril. People with dominant Kapha have a blunt nose and people with dominant Pitta have a sharp nostril.

Nail Diagnosis

Nails which can be dry and hard advocate a predominance of Vata constitution. Pink, smooth and easy nails are an example of Pitta charter. If the nails are robust, thick and really colourful, then Kapha predominates.

Lip Diagnosis (OSTHA)

Dry and difficult lips are an instance of vata imbalance. Repeated assaults of purple patches along the margins of the lips element in the path of a persistent pitta derangement.

Chapter 3: Hypertension and Ayurveda

Hypertension or immoderate blood pressure has become a number one reason of disability and demise all over the worldwide. If neglected, it may result in style of headaches like coronary coronary heart attacks, cerebrovascular stroke and kidney failure. In most cases, it does now not cause any obvious signs till those complications stand up. It performs the function of silent killer in the frame. Hence, it is critical to hold in mind that you could have hypertension and the first-rate manner you can recognize approximately it is to get your blood stress checked at everyday intervals.

What is excessive blood strain?

Hypertension method advanced pressure of the blood within the arteries. It is known as Rakta Gata Vata in Ayurveda. Normal blood stress of a healthful man or woman is a hundred and twenty mm of Hg systolic and eighty mm of Hg diastolic. The upward push in blood stress relies upon on the age, sex, own family statistics, bodily sports activities and weight loss program of someone.

Here are few Ayurvedic treatments which might be effective in reducing blood strain obviously:

Ashwagandha

Ashwagandha is a well-known Ayurvedic herb identified for its adaptogenic houses. It keeps the blood pressure interior ordinary limits and reduces contamination and damage inside the arteries added on because of the persistent excessive strain. It strengthens the mind and frame and improves the capacity of someone to cope with mental and bodily stress thereby tackling the idea reason of the contamination. It will also boom strength and resistance and produces a strengthening impact at the body capabilities.

Stress is one of the maximum normal reasons of immoderate blood strain. The immoderate production of pressure hormones like cortisol can result in further elevation of the blood stress. Ashwagandha growth the character's functionality to deal with stress thereby growing greater inner calmness. This, in flip, reduces the extent of cortisol circulating inside the frame and controls blood pressure.

Triphala

Triphala has been used due to the truth centuries for rejuvenating the frame. It includes three herbs that collectively form a effective mixture, which goes in a profound; however mild way. The 3 herbs are Haritaki (Terminalia chebula), Amla (Emblica officinalis) and Bibhitaki (Terminalia bellica).

Triphala reduces excessive blood strain and normalizes blood flow into. It moreover reduces ldl cholesterol, this is every other commonplace cause of high blood pressure and works towards preventing atherosclerosis. The anti-inflammatory and anti-weight problems effects of this device help in preventing hypertension via tackling the opportunity 2 causes of the contamination in particular infection and weight problems.

Jatamansi

Jatamansi protects the arteries from the damage due to free radicals. It upkeep the arterial harm because of ldl cholesterol plaques and thereby improves the internal diameter of the blood vessels. This lets in the blood to drift freely thru the arteries, which guarantees decrease pressure created through the use of the blood on the walls of arteries. This herb moreover creates a calming effect on the thoughts and frame and consequently, is surprisingly powerful in lowering mental stress.

Arjuna

Arjuna is a effective herb for treating immoderate blood stress. It reduces the quantity of low density lipoprotein (horrible) ldl cholesterol in the liver and increases the production of immoderate density lipoprotein (accurate) ldl ldl ldl cholesterol thereby lowering the risk of atherosclerosis.

It additionally reduces the effects of pressure and anxiety on the coronary heart through the use of lowering the producing of strain hormones and protects the blood vessels from the damage because of them.

These herbal treatments are based totally on the recovery concepts of Ayurveda. These herbs are regular and herbal and do now not cause any dangerous aspect effects.

Diet and Lifestyle recommendations

For better control of the contamination and for preventing the complications, patients are encouraged to study a few dietary and manner of life hints given underneath:

• Avoid meat and eggs. Reduce the consumption of table salt and one among a kind food items which might be immoderate in salt like pickles. Reduce protein intake. Eat loads of stop end result like melons and greens like Garlic, lemon and parsley.

• Avoid smoking because it will increase heart fee. Smoking moreover worsens atherosclerosis resulting in further aggravation of the hassle.

• Exercise often. Brisk on foot, strolling and swimming are top alternatives. Exercising additionally lets in to govern weight problems, that may be a common precursor of immoderate blood strain. Avoid strenuous sports activities if your blood pressure will be very excessive.

- Nurture love and affection. Love and an affectionate touch can drop your blood strain notably.

- Laughter is the great medicinal drug; it relieves anxiety and strain. It moreover emits first-rate power and lets in you keep terrible energies at bay. Laughter works as a amazing rest remedy additionally. It decreases the producing of strain hormones. If you are aggravated, irritated or unhappy; just chuckle and you could find out your self far from the style. It is a completely powerful remedy this is always with you, with out spending a penny for it.

Meditation and Breath Therapy for Hypertension:

You can gain entire tranquility of the mind through meditating in the Corpse Pose. To exercise this, take sluggish deep breaths and deliver interest to the incoming and outgoing breath. Focus on the temperature of the breath while breathing in and exhaling. You may be conscious that the inhaled air is slightly lots much less warmness than the exhaled air. Do this for 10 minutes day by day to get rid of strain and the ensuing immoderate blood strain. Research has proved that people, who workout Corpse Pose, frequently have a higher manipulate on their blood pressure.

Chapter 4: Diabetes and Ayurveda

Diabetes Mellitus

Diabetes Mellitus is a metabolic disorder, which impacts the capability of the body to make proper use of glucose. It might also arise because of the lack of Insulin produced within the pancreas (type 1 Diabetes) or due to the incapacity of the body to utilize the insulin correctly (Type 2 Diabetes). The danger elements for this circumstance encompass weight problems, sedentary life-style, family data, faulty weight loss plan and smoking. It is a chronic disorder characterized with the aid of continual excessive tiers of blood sugar because of the incorrect metabolism of carbohydrates in the frame. The greater of glucose in the blood moreover consequences in accelerated amount of glucose being handed in the urine. This motives an increase within the urine output due to which the patient moreover develops dehydration and elevated thirst.

Ayurvedic View

In Ayurveda, Diabetes Mellitus is referred to as Madhumeha. The phrase is derived from

Madhu, because of this 'honey' and Meha, which means 'urine'. This illness is assessed as Vataj Meha, an imbalance because of the greater of Vata or Air. Deterioration of the cells and tissues inside the frame is a characteristic characteristic of the impairment of Vata. This is the cause why all crucial organs which incorporates the liver, the coronary coronary coronary heart, the thoughts and the kidneys are affected due to Diabetes.

Madhumeha is taken into consideration a Maha Rog (Major Disease) because, if no longer dealt with nicely, it could reason crucial headaches like kidney failure, stroke, coronary coronary heart assaults and impotency. Though it's miles a metabolic ailment, it can't be managed by means of really reducing the sugar levels. Ayurveda recommends remedy that is geared toward rejuvenating the complete body except lowering the sugar degree. The holistic treatment additionally guarantees that no in addition complications are delivered about.

Natural control of Diabetes with herbs

There are severa herbs which may be notably powerful in decreasing the volume of sugar in blood. The finest advantage of these natural dietary supplements is that they purpose no side results even supposing used for severa years. Given under is a list of some of the most effective herbs for an powerful manage of Diabetes.

- Bitter Gourd

Bitter gourd is taken into consideration the wonderful herbal remedy for diabetes. Patients are advised to drink at least one tablespoon of bitter gourd juice every day. Alternatively, they also can upload 1 tablespoon of Indian gooseberry juice to at the least one cup of sour gourd juice and take this mixture every day. This will permit the pancreas to secrete more insulin.

- Cinnamon

Cinnamon enables alter blood sugar levels thru correcting the metabolism of carbohydrates in the frame. Research has discovered that this spice has the functionality to decrease the fasting blood glucose significantly. Regular use of Cinnamon in food schooling additionally enables to prevent any harm to the coronary heart and reduces the threat of coronary coronary heart attacks.

- Green Tea

Green tea includes polyphenols that possess strong antioxidant homes. The important antioxidant in green tea, Epigallocatechin Gallate (EGCG), has severa fitness benefits collectively with advanced glucose manipulate, higher insulin interest and faded threat of cardiac complications.

- Grapes

Many humans are surprised to realise that this juicy fruit can truly help in controlling diabetes. In fact; many patients assume they must keep away from this fruit. But, the fact is grapes encompass a chemical referred to as Resveratrol that enables in lowering blood sugar. It also can lessen highbrow pressure and lets in in preventing sudden upward thrust in blood sugar following disturbing situations.

- Garlic

Garlic or Allium Sativum gives strong antioxidant residences. The research have proved an instantaneous hyperlink the various everyday consumption of Garlic and an powerful control of diabetes. It motives a discount in blood glucose with the useful resource of developing the secretion of Insulin. It moreover slows down the degradation of insulin. The micro-circulatory results of this herb help in improving the float of blood within the vital organs of the body thereby preventing the complications because of the shortage of blood supply like stroke and peripheral vascular problems.

- Bauhinia Forficata

Bauhinia Forficata has been known as 'vegetable insulin' due to the brilliant recuperation effect it produces in patients laid low with Type 1 Diabetes. Regular usage of this herb as tea infusion can assist sufferers keep the disorder on top of things.

- Ivy gourd

Ivy gourd or Coccinia Indica has been located to very own insulin-mimetic homes, due to this it mimics the motion of insulin. It also allows glucose uptake through the body so that it may be used as an power source. Significant favorable adjustments in blood sugar degree have been discovered in research concerning this herb. Some studies have furthermore referred to regeneration of the islet cells (the pancreatic cells that modify the carbohydrate metabolism) and an boom in beta-cellular hobby.

- Milk Thistle

Milk Thistle or Silibum Marianum consists of excessive concentrations of antioxidants and flavonoids, that have a useful effect on insulin resistance. It improves the receptivity of the frame cells to insulin and makes it extra powerful. It is broadly used inside the treatment of Type 2 Diabetes.

Diet and manner of lifestyles adjustments for Diabetes

The Ayurvedic remedy for this illness is based at the complete exchange within the way of life of the person. Along with herbal tablets, sufferers also are advocated to consume nutritious food and lead a healthy way of life. Lifestyle and dietary modifications rejuvenate the cells and tissues within the body, allowing them to produce extra insulin.

Here are a few nutritional pointers for diabetic patients. These guidelines also can help prevent the superiority of the illness in parents which is probably inside the excessive-threat category.

- Avoid sugar in any shape which includes rice, potato, cereals and stop result like mangoes, pineapple and banana

- Include one bitter dish in at least one meal of a day

- Eat masses of black gram, inexperienced vegetables, fish and soy

- Eat vegetables like string beans, cucumber, bitter gourd, onion and garlic and end result like Jambul and watermelon

Lifestyle for Diabetes sufferers

- Quit smoking

- Avoid slumbering for the duration of daylight

- Exercise frequently

- Control your weight

- Take good enough eye care

- Take more care of your foot

Chapter 5: Treatment and technique of Ayurveda for ldl cholesterol issues

What is hypercholesterolemia?

Hypercholesterolemia is a illness characterised by means of excessive stage of ldl ldl ldl cholesterol. Cholesterol is a mild, waxy substance placed some of the fat in all of the frame's cells, mainly in the bloodstream. It is positioned in small quantities and office work a part of the nerve coverings, cell walls and the mind cells. Hence, it has an critical feature inside the body. However, at the same time as this substance is determined in excess quantities, it may motive blockages within the arteries resulting in extreme effects.

Ayurvedic treatment for dealing with ldl ldl cholesterol problems

Ayurvedic technique for treating this situation includes getting rid of the pollution and mucus from the blood vessels and to repair the digestive hearth to allow it to perform optimally for burning greater fats.

Dangers of excessive cholesterol

Excessive amount of ldl cholesterol circulating inside the blood can result in a slow increase of this substance inside the walls of the arteries of the coronary heart and thoughts. It combines with special substances and forms thick, tough deposits known as plaque that could clog the ones arteries. This circumstance is called atherosclerosis. If the plaque breaks away in piece and circulates in blood, it is able to journey to remote organs similar to the coronary heart or the mind inflicting coronary heart attacks or stroke, respectively. Here are a few herbs that have robust medicinal homes for decreasing ldl ldl ldl cholesterol:

- Alfalfa

Alfalfa clears the arteries congested with ldl ldl cholesterol thru generating a disintegrating impact on the plaques. Regular consumption of this herb can help people manage their cholesterol levels and keep away from the complications of this example.

- Arjuna

Arjuna has been used thinking about the fact that centuries in the manipulate of cardiac issues like coronary coronary heart attacks. The bark of this herb, at the same time as taken in a powder shape, has useful medicinal houses. It can dissolve the ldl ldl cholesterol collected inside the coronary arteries and reduces the hazard of coronary heart assaults.

- Coriander

Coriander works as an notable diuretic. It enables to control ldl ldl cholesterol by using manner of boosting the skills of the kidneys. It ensures that the kidneys flush out the greater cholesterol from the body thru urine thereby reducing blood ldl ldl cholesterol degree.

- Garlic

Garlic is fairly useful for humans with ldl ldl cholesterol problems. Experts endorse ingesting to three cloves of garlic regular, first thing within the morning. It can be chewed uncooked if the sharp taste can be tolerated or certainly gulped down with a tumbler of water. It allows to get rid of the ldl ldl cholesterol from the blood thru disintegrating the plaques and frees up the arteries.

● Guggulu

This is a famous Indian herb, which has robust medicinal homes for treating ldl cholesterol-related coronary heart troubles. It includes guggulsterones that help reduce the cholesterol levels. It also has the capacity to dissolve the ldl ldl cholesterol plaques in the arteries just so it can be excreted thru urine.

Dietary and life-style adjustments for handling excessive ldl ldl ldl cholesterol

Ayurveda moreover shows a disciplined healthy eating plan and ordinary exercise plan to gain wholesome levels of cholesterol. Here are a while-tested measures that would help patients bring their levels of cholesterol to normal and keep it that manner.

● Start your day with immoderate fiber grains like oats and easy give up cease result. Eat hundreds of dried beans or legumes and seafood mainly salmon, sardine and tuna. Oysters, mussels and clams also are beneficial in reducing ldl cholesterol.

- Eat hundreds of culmination centered in antioxidant compounds like citrus end result, apple and strawberries. Nuts like almonds and walnut and veggies like spinach, broccoli and carrots also are wealthy in antioxidant compounds.

- Drink loads of water. This reasons an multiplied excretion of water alongside facet the pollution and excess fats from the body.

- Do everyday carrying sports activities like brisk on foot - for at the least 40 minutes everyday, for five days in keeping with week. Regular bodily activities can assist control weight troubles and enhance the frame's metabolic fee, which, in turn, accelerates using excess fats.

- Keep an eye constant on the quantity of calories you eat. Say no to crimson meats, sweets, ice creams and all outstanding materials that would increase your calorie do not forget. Foods wealthy in fat like fried components, too, should be prevented.

- Practice deep breathing workout and meditation for 15-20 minutes every day. It lets in refresh your mind and body and is likewise an powerful de-pressure approach.

• Quit smoking. Smoking will increase the tendency for the blood to clot and worsens atherosclerosis. It moreover motives damage to the partitions of the arteries. Besides this, the recuperation of patients, who have suffered a coronary coronary heart assault because of immoderate ldl ldl cholesterol, is a lot slower in folks that smoke than in nonsmokers.

• Avoid extra of alcohol. People, who devour slight amounts of alcohol, have a lower threat of cardiac headaches than non-drinkers. However, advanced consumption of alcohol can result in other health risks like immoderate blood strain, stroke and weight issues.

Chapter 6: Skin Care in Ayurveda

Skin is the most important revel in organ of our frame. It is likewise the a part of the body that defines the splendor and splendor of a person and a girl. Skin serves as a protecting barrier among our internal organs and safeguards it from any damage due to the elements inside the out of doors environment. Skin regulates the frame temperature and is in a non-stop state of boom, with antique cells death and the brand new cells forming. The skin is tormented by every issue of our life, which embody what we eat, even as and what form of we sleep and wherein we stay.

Why is pores and pores and skin care vital?

Proper pores and skin care is essential for all men and women who are worried approximately their physical appearance. Unhealthy pores and skin seems silly, at the same time as a wholesome pores and pores and skin appears colorful and glowing. Wrinkles boom with extra ease if your pores and skin is terrible and not nicely hydrated. An horrific pores and skin additionally loses its elasticity faster and makes it sag and expand folds. A healthful pores and skin has an potential to heal faster. Therefore, it's miles essential to take right care of your pores and skin truly so it seems radiant and exudes self belief on your personality.

Ayurvedic method for pores and skin care

The holistic manipulate of skin troubles in ayurveda carries of the 3-fold approach through herbal medicinal capsules, food regimen and life-style.

Ayurveda has stated that pores and pores and pores and skin issues within the essential arise because of the sluggish liver features resulting in Kapha and Pitta Dosha. It reasons a building up of pollution inside the body and later the ones impurities display up as pores and pores and skin issues like spoil-outs, eczema or pigmentations. Ayurveda advises humans to drink loads of water to flush out the impurities.

Another vital detail that could make contributions to the healthful appearance of the pores and pores and skin is a clean bowel.

Ayurveda stresses on the want for regular and entire evacuation of the bowels. In order to acquire this, a weight-reduction plan excessive in fibers like papaya, oranges and watermelons is usually recommended.

Stress is the maximum not unusual reason of pores and pores and skin problems. The prevalence or aggravation of pimples, eczema, melasma and pores and skin most cancers is largely connected to highbrow stress. It starts a chain of reaction resulting in dryness of the pores and pores and skin, lack of pores and pores and skin luster and wrinkle formation. Ayurveda advises human beings to take a look at the de-stressing techniques like yoga, meditation and deep respiratory physical sports activities for maintaining the pores and skin extra younger and more healthful.

The 3 superb herbs for an appealing and colourful pores and pores and skin

1. Turmeric (Haldi)

Turmeric nourishes the pores and skin, purifies blood and offers it a natural glow. It

42

possesses anti-growing older, anti-inflammatory and anti-bacterial residences that assist lessen infection in zits, pigmentations and blemishes and forestalls infections. It also heals ulcers and wounds at the pores and skin. It is idea for its hydrating homes. It prevents dryness of the pores and pores and skin and continues it soft and supple. It additionally slows down the pores and skin developing older device.

How to Use:

• On a warm day, blend 2 spoonfuls of turmeric powder in half of the amount of rice powder, tomato juice and uncooked milk every to make a paste. Apply it on the face and neck and leave it for 1/2-hour. Rinse with lukewarm water. The pores and pores and pores and skin will appearance brighter and sparkling after this.

• You also can use it as a night time time cream. Prepare a paste from turmeric and yogurt or milk and observe it on your face. Leave it on in a single day and wash off the masks gently within the morning with water.

- Apply a mixture of turmeric and lime juice on the exposed areas of the pores and pores and pores and skin to remove tanning.

2. Sandalwood (Chandan)

Sandalwood is the critical factor difficulty in maximum of the Ayurvedic skin-care components. It is effective in treating rashes, scrapes, zits and blemishes. The paste and oil of Sandalwood, whilst used externally, produce a groovy, calming effect at the body. It lets in balance the frame after overexposure to the sun and prevents sunburns. Sandalwood powder can be made into a paste for hydrating and cleansing the pores and skin.

How to Use:

- To address acne, make a thick paste of 1 teaspoon of sandalwood powder and 1 teaspoon of turmeric. Apply the paste on the zits earlier than going to mattress.

- You can deal with eczema with the aid of way of making use of the aggregate of sandalwood and lime juice on the affected additives. Leave it for 20-half of-hour and rinse with cool water. This will assist lessen the itching and irritation of the pores and pores and pores and skin.

• Sandalwood oil is used as a moisturizer for the face. Gentle rub down of the face and the frame with this oil could have a rejuvenating effect at the pores and pores and skin. It moreover relaxes the muscles and makes one sense lighter; but energetic.

• Mix four teaspoons of sandalwood powder in teaspoons of almond oil and 5 tablespoons of coconut oil. Apply this mixture on the uncovered elements of your pores and pores and skin. You will word a large development for your tan.

three.   Aloe Vera (Ghritkumari)

Aloe Vera is a well-known ayurvedic medicinal drug stated for its anti inflammatory and anti-fungal homes. It also possesses restoration and cooling houses. It hastens the restoration of pimples, pores and pores and skin wounds, burns, scalds, insect bites, blisters and rashes. It is likewise used for alleviating the signs of allergic reactions of the pores and pores and skin and vaginal contamination. The gel of this plant can protect the outer layer of the pores and pores and pores and skin and prevent irritation.

How to use:

• Apply Aloe Vera gel on the face in advance than utilizing any make-up. This will assist save you the pores and pores and skin from drying.

• Add the pulp of some smooth culmination to Aloe Vera gel and located this in a blender to make a thick paste. Use it as a face % to keep the skin cool.

• Mix Aloe Vera with almond oil or wheat germ and use it as a moisturizing p.C..

• To cope with pigmentation, lessen a leaf of Aloe Vera and split it to remove the gel. Apply the gel on the pores and pores and pores and skin and depart it for 10-20 mins. Wash it off with slight cleansing cleaning soap and water.

Chapter 7: Medicinal utilization of herbs & spices - your kitchen pharmacy

In a first rate international, we're able to get all the vitamins we want from the food we consume. But regrettably we do no longer live in a splendid international. The food to be had to us has surpassed via a drastic change inside the beyond century, making wholesome eating a mission. We normally have a tendency to devour extra of horrible or junk food than nutritious and healthy food although we have got our spice rack packed with seasonings having wonderful medicinal powers. We without a doubt draw close the ones spices in a hurry, but can we apprehend the recuperation powers those historical herbs very own? Do we apprehend that, at the identical time as used frequently and inside the proper manner, the ones kitchen spices and herbs can in truth turn our kitchen right right into a pharmacy that has a remedy for most fitness troubles?

Much earlier than the fitness stores made precise herbs without a doubt to be had for restoration use, humans relied on these culinary herbs to play a pharmaceutical feature inside the circle of relatives.

The super aspect about the ones spices and herbs is that most oldsters have already got them in our kitchen, which makes the complete manner masses much less intimidating.

Using kitchen herbs is heaps an awful lot less pricey and does now not require an in depth knowledge of herbal remedy. Anyone can use the ones herbs correctly to heal and regenerate the frame. Before you start to take a inventory of your spice rack, permit's discover approximately the commonplace culinary herbs and spices, a manner to apply them and their restoration homes.

Basil

Basil produces a strong antimicrobial and antioxidant interest. It stimulates the urge for meals and eases stomach upsets. Basil allows the kidney skills and permits in detoxifying the blood thru disposing of the damaging pollutants from the body via urine. Basil also sharpens reminiscence and improves interest span and awareness strength. It eases gum ulcers, earaches and itching or infection of the pores and skin. Use Basil leaves in soups, salads and dips. You can also saute it with greens or use it in pasta sauces.

Ginger

Ginger has anti inflammatory homes that shield the frame in competition to infections as a result of bacteria and fungi. It furthermore gets rid of intestinal gas and soothes the intestinal tract, at the identical time as boosting the immune machine. It can prevent the progression of atherosclerosis through decreasing levels of cholesterol. Ginger moreover allows to triumph over nausea. Ginger may be lessen into smaller portions and taken to any food guidance.

Nutmeg

Nutmeg is used to reinforce highbrow fitness and to reduce tension. It elicits a considerable antidepressant-like impact this is similar to the antidepressants like Imipramine and Fluoxetine. It additionally may be used for treating insomnia, restlessness and anxiety.

Cloves

Clove is one of the pleasant stimulants. It is concept for its vaso-exciting houses. Cloves are wealthy in minerals like iron, calcium, sodium, potassium and manganese. Clove oil may be used as a community anesthetic agent for alleviating toothache. It additionally reduces cough, allergic reactions, bronchitis and stress.

Cinnamon

Cinnamon contains calcium, iron and manganese. It can be used inside the remedy of dietary deficiencies like anemia. Cinnamon may be utilized by diabetic sufferers to control their blood sugar tiers. It reduces digestive problems and improves mind abilties.

Parsley

Parsley's medicinal effects come from its flavonoids: apiole, terpinolene, myristicin and appin. Parsley gives healing benefits within the manage of renal problems like urinary tract infections and kidney stones. It is likewise effective in relieving gastrointestinal misery. Moreover, it can additionally be used to regularize menses. Use it in salads or soups as a garnish. Take care now not to overcook it because the herb also can lose its efficiency and shade.

Bay Leaf

Bay leaf acts as a stimulant for the pores and pores and pores and skin. It improves the glow on the skin and makes it greater agency and mild thereby preventing wrinkles. Regular use of this herb in food can assist prevent rashes in patients having a sensitive pores and pores and skin. Use it as a flavoring agent for stews, soups, pilafs and with seafood.

Tarragon

Tarragon works well as a de-worming agent. Parents can supply this herb to their youngsters to stave off intestinal parasites. Tarragon has additionally been used to address toothaches and gastric upsets. Just like parsley, Tarragon also can be used to manipulate menstrual troubles like amenorrhea and dysmenorrhea. It is carried out in traditional French sauces, vinegars and vinaigrettes. It moreover may be used to roast fowl.

Dill

Dill is used to address gastrointestinal troubles like stomach disillusioned, flatulence, gastric ulcers and indigestion. It is also used to deal with insomnia, stress and tension disorders. Some parents provide an infusion or tea of Dill to their younger infants for relieving colic. Dill is used inside the guidance of pickles, fish stews and beet soups.

Lavender

Lavender is an extraordinary ayurvedic treatment for treating loss of urge for meals and insomnia. It is determined to be useful inside the treatment of circulatory problems. It is frequently used to deal with migraine, restlessness and cramps. Lavender can be utilized in teas, scones, cookies and candies. It may be blended with honey, mint, oats or rose syrup for including flavor.

Oregano

Oregano allows in the remedy of breathing illnesses like stuffy nose and persistent cough. It works as an expectorant. It liquefies the secretions and aids within the clean expulsion of the mucus thereby relieving respiration troubles delivered about due to the blockages. It is robust in relieving menstrual cramping and has effective antimicrobial sports activities activities. Oregano can be used to taste olive oil and to season lamb and goat milk cheeses. It is likewise utilized in tomato sauces and in chilies.

Sage

Sage is concept for its recovery houses for easing infection, in particular of the mouth. It improves appetite and eases digestion. Nursing mothers, who experience overproduction of the milk resulting in breast engorgement, can use Sage to gradual the milk manufacturing. This herb is used as a rub for red meat and to roast chook.

Rosemary

Rosemary is used to ease headaches and migraines. It additionally allows to alleviate belly upsets and menstrual problems. It may be applied externally to rush the restoration of wounds and eczema. Rosemary also can help lower blood stress in patients with hypertension. Rosemary is applied in herbal vinegars and roasts.

Peppermint

Peppermint is usually taken as a tea or in infusions to address colic and digestive disenchanted. It is usually used in the remedy of commonplace cold and flu, manner to its capability to open the sinuses. When utilized in aggregate with honey, it can help ease a sore throat. Peppermint crucial oil may be carried out at the temples to assist with complications and migraines. It is utilized in chocolates and confections. It additionally may be used inside the steerage of whipped cream or fruit salad and as a garnishment to roast lamb.

Licorice

Licorice boosts the immune device and buffers the inflammatory reaction through stimulating the manufacturing of steroids via the usage of the adrenal glands. It moreover modifies the reaction of the immune tool to combat and relieve the signs and symptoms and symptoms and signs and symptoms of contamination.

Chapter 8: The Ayurvedic First Aid Kit
contamination.

Children in addition to adults are at risk of incidents that would harm us or even bring about minor or essential injuries. So, all and sundry preserve a number one beneficial aid package organized at domestic complete of bandages, antiseptic cream, plasters, wipes, pain killing tablets and antacids. But, what in case you want to obtain a brief first aid comfort without a doubt? With just a little patience and right recognize how, you may without trouble discover a herbal remedy out of your private kitchen for administering first beneficial aid in case of emergencies. Here are few first useful resource natural treatments that you may use in such case:

Sore throat

A traditional mixture of turmeric and honey works rapid and correctly for easing a sore throat. Just blend a spoonful of each those natural remedies and suck on the spoon. Alternatively, you could upload turmeric and rock salt in heat water and do gargling. You will find a right away consolation from the hassle.

Cuts

Applying a paste of turmeric and honey at the lessen will prevent the bleeding inside few seconds. Just make the paste and press it at the wound. It also acts as an anti-septic and prevents any contamination. It may additionally even help the wound to heal quicker. This natural tip is useful even for diabetic sufferers in whom any harm can take an extended time to heal and might bring about an contamination.

Burn

The first thing to do in case of burns is to proper away run the component through bloodless water. Let the water float over the detail as long as the burning sensation stays. This will not best relieve the ache; however moreover save you the blisters from forming. Then, exercise a paste of Aloe Vera gel with a pinch of turmeric powder. You can go away it until the initial sting subsides. You can keep using aloe or exercise coconut oil with sandalwood or rose to enhance the cooling effect.

Headache

Apply a paste of ginger on the forehead and lie down for about 5-10 minutes. Then, eliminate the paste. You will locate the headache disappearing miraculously after this. The aroma of Ginger may even make you sense extra refreshed. Headaches moreover may be a signal of dehydration. So, drink 1-2 glasses of water in particular in case you start getting headache after a workout or due to journeying below harsh solar. A mild rubdown to the forehead, temples, shoulders and neck with Eucalyptus oil can also help loosen up the muscle agencies and relieve the headache. Sinus headache can be relieved with the useful resource of utilizing gingelly oil combined with camphor on the brow.

Acid reflux

Acid reflux is usually a result of an boom in the pitta dosha. A pitta pacifying healthy eating plan can help accurate this hassle fast. You can attempt chewing on fennel seeds or drink Aloe Vera juice to relieve the ache. You can also drink a glass of buttermilk with a pinch of fenugreek and asafetida. This will help neutralize the acid within the stomach and prevent regurgitation and the following heartburn.

Indigestion

The nice herbal brief recuperation for this very common hassle is consuming a glass of pomegranate juice. You also can attempt drinking warmth water infused with lemon juice. Drinking buttermilk with cumin seeds and a hint salt can assist relieve flatulence and stomach ache right now.

Cold and Cough

Dry cough can be treated through taking a decoction of liquorice root. If you be laid low with manner of cough with lot of mucous secretion, take a decoction of ginger, turmeric, pinch of black pepper, lemon and a squeeze of honey as speedy because it cools down. You can also consume a paste of garlic or chunk on ginger root. You will discover exquisite comfort through boiling some ginger powder in water and breathing within the steam. Applying few drops of Eucalyptus oil on the edges of the nose will assist to relieve nose block. Inhaling the powder of calamus root into each nose also can reduce the congestion.

Diarrhea

If diarrhea is a cease result of indigestion or overeating, drink a glass of buttermilk with a pinch of salt and asafetida. Another super remedy for treating unfastened motions is powdered mango seed excited about honey. A blend of rock salt, dry ginger and jaggery is likewise effective in times of diarrhea due to indigestion.

Acne

Acne may be an emergency once in a while. A small pimple proper here or there in your face can ship you in a tizzy specifically when it plants up in advance than a completely unique event. Though the pimple will not disappear virtually inner handiest a day, it could lessen extensive and seem a good deal much less visible thru the usage of utilising a paste of sandalwood powder and turmeric on it. Take approximately one teaspoon of every of these powders and blend them with rose water to make a paste. For internal remedy, drink 1 cup of sparkling Aloe vera juice, times a day, until the zits clears.

Asthma

Combine ginger herb with Licorice and drink it as a tea. The encouraged share is about one teaspoon of every the herbs for one cup of water. Drinking onion juice combined with 1-2 teaspoons of honey and a pinch of black pepper can also offer treatment from allergies assault.

Backache

Gentle rubdown of the again with a paste of ginger and eucalyptus oil can assist relieve the spasm of the muscle mass inside the again and decrease once more ache. Backache due to bone-associated issues can be relieved by using way of massaging with coconut oil. However, it may simplest reduce the pain for a quick period and now not treatment the disease really.

Bad breath

Drinking half of a cup of Aloe Vera and eating a teaspoonful of fennel seeds can assist lessen the lousy breath. You also can chunk on peppermint or ginger to keep away from this hassle.

Bleeding

External bleeding may be arrested by manner of using utilising ice or sandalwood paste. For preventing inner bleeding, patients are counseled to drink heat milk with half of of teaspoon every of saffron and turmeric powder. This ought to be observed through session with a systematic professional to have a observe the purpose of bleeding just so appropriate measures may be taken.

Toothache

Toothache may be straight away relieved through making use of 2-three drops of clove oil on the affected tooth. You also can located the drops on a piece of sterilized cotton ball and press it among the tooth. Gargling with salt water or slightly heat sesame oil also can offer treatment from toothache.

Boils

Applying a paste of ginger and turmeric powder straight away on the boil or using cooked onions as a poultice can assist a boil heal rapid.

Burning in the Eyes

Put in four drops of rose water or clean Aloe Vera juice into the affected eye. You can also have a look at Castor oil to the soles of the toes.

Chapter 9: Food antidotes in Ayurveda

What is antidote?

An antidote is a substance that counteracts a particular remedy or an unpleasant sensation. Sometimes, the meals we consume can purpose many troubles like nausea, vomiting, diarrhea, gastric hassle, pores and skin rashes and allergic reactions. These bad results can arise because of overindulgence or hypersensitivity of the person to that substance.

While it's far right to keep away from overindulging too often, it is tough to provide away the temptation and 'permit our hair down' from time to time. Besides meals gadgets, there are various specific elements like excessive publicity to the solar and traveling that would have an impact on our will being and eventually, need to be tackled effectively. You can counter the horrible outcomes of these things with the resource of the use of the herbal herbs in ayurveda. Below I've listed some powerful, natural antidotes that you may use to offset the 'no longer so wholesome' results of positive subjects.

Overindulgences & Their antidotes:

Chocolate

In Ayurveda, chocolate is a conventional instance of 'Srota Blocker'. Srotas are the 'channels' within the body that want to be stored clean if you want to make sure extremely good health and power. When those channels are blocked, they motive unpleasant symptoms and signs and signs or even maximum vital illnesses. The predominant culprits in chocolate are the immoderate diploma of carbohydrates and milk solids. You can counter the terrible impact of goodies through the use of consuming warm water with cardamom pods. The warm water enables 'melt' the improperly digested foodstuffs and cardamom pods re-open the srotas or channels.

Alcohol

The worst impact of excessive alcohol intake is at the liver cells. Alcohol can produce an terrible impact at the liver capabilities ensuing in hepatitis, alcoholic liver sickness, ascites and subsequently liver most cancers. Though the impact cannot be reversed genuinely, a superb cut rate within the alcoholic liver harm can be achieved through the intake of turmeric. People are recommended to take 1-2 pinches of this herb in a glass of water or add it to regular cooking as part of preferred regular.

Drinking warm water with a pinch of turmeric also can offer consolation from hangover. The stimulating and depressing outcomes of alcohol can be prevented through the usage of consuming 1-2 cardamom seeds or chewing a pinch of cumin seeds. Another herb that could assist address hangover is dried out Ojas. Ojas improves digestion and is notion to be the primary link amongst attention and our frame. It is taken into consideration the fabric equal of bliss and gives us mental readability and resistance to sickness.

Seafood

Seafood is 'warm' by using way of manner of nature and might reason problems related to digestive warmth like heartburn, acid reflux disorder disorder ailment, gastritis and indigestion. The terrific antidote to offset the effect of seafood is Peppermint Tea. It reduces the greater belly warm temperature and forestalls the ugly signs and signs and symptoms and signs. I assume that is in which the tradition of ingesting 'peppermint' after dinner came from… although it's tough to provide an explanation for wherein the chocolate got here into the equation!!!

Sunburn

The first rate antidote to relieve the symptoms and signs and signs of sunburn is Aloe Vera. Fresh Aloe Vera gel is enormously therapeutic for a sun-broken pores and skin. Apply regularly to save you pores and pores and skin damage and hasten restore.

Red eyes

Soreness or redness of the eyes can stand up due to a number of reasons which incorporates infections, solar exposure and overuse. An effective and time-tested antidote for the sore eyes brought approximately due to the exposure to solar is rose water eye spray. Add 2-3 spoons of rose water in a pitcher of water and splash it on the eyes or eye bathtub with cold milk. Putting sliced cucumbers on each the eyelids can also counter the effect of harsh solar on the eyes.

Motion illness

Ayurveda recommends glowing ginger squeeze for decreasing motion illness. Take 1/4th teaspoon of freshly squeezed ginger juice and upload to it a hint lemon juice and a pinch of salt. Simply lick the spoon dipped in this mixture to eliminate the sensation. Coffee

Most human beings will be surprised to understand that immoderate intake of coffee can cause unsightly signs and symptoms. Coffee carries caffeine, which over-stimulates the worried device ensuing in insomnia. Drinking a pitcher of warmth milk or 2-3 glasses of warm water will counter the impact of greater caffeine for your body and could assist you get a great sleep. The sick-results of espresso moreover can be stored at bay through the usage of nutmeg powder.

Besides those, there are numerous one of a kind substances like cheese, eggs, curd, fish and meat that would purpose a horrible effect on our body. Since the negative results of those food gadgets are acknowledged, you may cause them to healthful by way of the usage of way of mixing them with the proper counteracting food gadgets or "antidotes" as given below:

• Cheese increases mucous production and congestion in the respiration passages ensuing in nostril block and breathlessness. It furthermore aggravates pitta and kapha. You can counteract this effect with the useful resource of along with black pepper to it.

• Eggs, in uncooked form, can growth kapha and in cooked shape, can increase pitta. Counter this via using including turmeric or by manner of manner of consuming uncooked onions with them.

• Ice-cream can cause severe breathing problems and nasal congestion. If taking ice-cream is inevitable, pinnacle it with cardamom and clove.

- Curd is also recognized to increase the mucous production and motive nasal congestion. Using cumin and ginger let you address the unwell-results of curd.

- Legumes are identified to offer gaseous distention of the stomach. Garlic, black pepper, cloves, ginger and chili powder are the high-quality antidotes for this.

- Fish can increase pitta. Lime, coconut and lemon are the satisfactory remedial measures to antidote the terrible results of fish.

Chapter 10: Yoga and Ayurveda

Yoga is an ancient technological know-how that targets at balancing the mind for attaining self-hobby and attention. It famous to us the decision of the sport powers of the frame, thoughts, breath and the senses. It furthermore unfolds the transformational strategies to paintings on them thru herbs, asana, eating regimen, pranayama and meditation. Yoga has the energy to alternate the lives of individuals who exercise it regularly. Ayurveda and yoga artwork collectively for maximum suited health and strength.

Link amongst Yoga and ayurveda

It is quite a revelation to appearance how ayurveda and yoga are interrelated. Both originate from a greater gadget of Vedic understanding that we are in a role to name as our nurturing mother. Ayurveda originates inside the Atharva Veda and Rig Veda and Yoga originates within the Yajur Veda.

Just like ayurveda, the ideas of yoga also are based totally totally on the requirements of the panchamahabuthas (earth, region, fireplace, air, water) and trigunas (sattva, rajas and tamas). Yoga and ayurveda encompass an knowledge of techniques our body works and the impact of meals and drugs on our frame.

In remedy, ayurveda and yoga each endorse a ordinary exercising of pranayama and meditation together with using herbs, following wholesome diet, body purification techniques and chanting of mantras for better bodily and mental fitness.

You can gain from practising a chain of yoga posture to remedy the most immoderate shape of dosha (kapha, vata, pitta) for your body. This will can help you restore your frame to a extra balanced, serene us of a.

What are the advantages of Yoga?

Peaceful mind, appropriate fitness, weight reduction, a sturdy and flexible frame and a glowing lovely pores and pores and skin– a few element you will be looking for, yoga will let you advantage it. Yoga isn't always restrained to asanas (yoga poses). Its benefits may be perceived not handiest at the bodily stage; but furthermore in uniting the thoughts, body and breath. When your body is in concord with the mind and soul, the adventure through life turns into a top notch deal happier, calmer and more pleasurable.

- All-round fitness

A accurate fitness does not recommend mere absence of a disorder. It is a satisfied, loving and enthusiastic expression of lifestyles. Yoga will let you stay physical healthful and emotionally balanced. The postures, meditation and pranayama (breathing strategies) of yoga together provide a holistic fitness bundle deal.

- Weight loss

Obesity is a totally commonplace health trouble that has most variety of medicinal drugs, which promise instantaneous brilliant outcomes. However, humans who've tried them understand that weight reduction can't be finished via the ones so-referred to as 'magic' tablets. However, weight loss plan - some one-of-a-kind commonplace approach to weight loss - isn't an smooth approach to stick to for a long time. People will be inclined to provide in to their temptations and start binge ingesting simply indoors some days of beginning their crash weight-reduction plan over-enthusiastically. Crash eating regimen and using 'magic' pills can also have severa terrible consequences at the health. On the possibility hand, Yoga offers slow weight reduction in a natural and healthful manner. Kapal Bhati pranayama and Sun Salutations (Surya Namaskar) are some techniques to shed pounds with yoga. Regular workout of yoga can also help us emerge as greater sensitive to the form of meals our body dreams and while. This can help us to hold a take a look at at the weight gain in destiny.

- Stress relief

Practicing yoga for a couple of minutes throughout the day is a extremely good way to remove pressure. Yoga postures, meditation and pranayama are the only techniques for releasing highbrow anxieties and physical strain.

- Inner peace

We often plan to visit serene spots, rich in herbal splendor to achieve the internal peace. However, we do not recognize that peace can also be located proper inner us. We can take our mini-excursion to enjoy serenity any time of the day! You can achieve the benefits of a small excursion everyday with yoga. It enables calm a disturbed mind.

- Improved immunity

Our device is a combination of mind, spirit and frame. Any unpleasantness or restlessness within the thoughts can take area as a physical contamination and any irregularity in the body could have an effect at the mind. Yoga poses red meat up the muscle tissues, manage restlessness and enhance the immunity thereby stopping such irregularities.

- Living with greater hobby

Our thoughts is continuously concerned in a unmarried or the other interest. It maintains swinging from the beyond to the destiny; but in no way remains inside the gift. We can shop ourselves from getting labored up and relax the mind thru being privy to this tendency of the mind. Yoga permits us create that awareness and brings the mind returned to the existing, wherein it can stay targeted.

- Better relationships

Yoga assist you to beautify the connection together in conjunction with your parents, spouse, friends and loved ones! A snug, satisfied and contented mind is better able to address sensitive relationship issues.

- Increased energy

We need to preserve shuttling among more than one obligations in the direction of the day. Due to this, we revel in genuinely drained out with the aid of the give up of the day. A few minutes of yoga can find out the secrets and techniques to feeling sparkling and active after an extended, tiring day. A 10-minute meditation at the same time as at table will let you experience recharged in the middle of a hectic day.

- Better posture and flexibility

Including yoga in our every day everyday can benefit the frame to grow to be flexible and supple. Regular yoga tones and stretches the frame muscle mass and makes them strong. It moreover improves the body posture while you stand, sit down or walk. This, in turn, will let you do away with the ailments added approximately due to wrong posture.

- Better intuition

Yoga has the energy to enhance your intuitive functionality so that you can effects understand what wants to be finished, how and while, to yield remarkable outcomes.

The Vedic device of drugs (Ayurveda) and the Vedic spiritual exercise (Yoga) together form a entire approach to deliver concord and properly-being to the mind, body and soul. Yoga is a non-stop method. The extra ordinary you're on the aspect of your yoga practice, the extra profound are its advantages. So, keep schooling!

Chapter 11: Massage remedies in Ayurveda

Ayurvedic rubdown creates a deep rest inside the muscle corporations of the frame and corrects the deeply rooted imbalances in the device thereby restoring concord and practical integrity of the doshas. Ayurvedic massage uses unique types of medicated oils for inducing prolonged, lively strokes in the course of the body.

Ayurveda offers rubdown treatment alternatives that motive at maintaining the enzymes inside the body at their normal functioning degree, thereby revitalizing the tissues and cells. A rub down allows soothe the nerves and strengthens the bones. It furthermore creates a enjoy of tranquility within the mind, delays the tool of having vintage and reduces the danger of destiny illnesses.

Some extra benefits of Ayurvedic Massage Therapies encompass:

• Improves blood circulate and lymphatic drainage

• Eliminates pollution from the frame

- Alleviates functionality destructive results of pressure

- Stimulates the immune electricity and strengthens the resistance to infections

- Eases constipation, relieves belly spasm and aids in digestion

- Eases muscular aches and pains whilst promoting muscle relaxation

Here are some rub down recovery techniques provided in ayurveda

- Abhyangam

Abhyangam is characterised via the usage of manner of lengthy strokes, Marma aspect remedy and flowing movements. Abhyangam is a high-priced, warmth oil rub down that focuses on calming the circulatory and nervous systems. This whole frame rub down improves the functionality of vitamins to acquire all the frame cells and gets rid of the stagnant waste. Concoction of heat natural oils used on this rub down nourishes and revitalizes the tissues. It heightens awareness and directs the internal recuperation gadget of the body. This remedy produces a deep restoration effect through the use of bringing concord into the body, mind and spirit, naturally. Abhyangam is an terrific clearly happy enjoy.

- Udwartanam (Herbal Anti-cellulite remedy)

Udwartanam is one of the most rejuvenating and a laugh remedies in Ayurveda. The simple gadget includes massaging the whole frame under the neckline. It uses a powder prepared from an series of herbs inside the course contrary to the hair increase. It opens the circulatory channels and permits metabolic hobby. It moreover improves the complexion of the skin and is fairly effective in reducing extra fats from the frame.

- Shirodhara

Shirodhara awakens the thoughts on the equal time as lulling the entire body to create a nation of calmness. Stimulation and rub down of the Marma elements on the pinnacle, shoulders, neck and the ft is observed through warm streams of Ayurvedic oil poured on and during the brow, usually. A deep intuitive and meditative nation is awakened and a fantastic intellectual clarity and shift of focus is professional at a few degree inside the treatment. Shirodhara releases pressure and quiets the thoughts. In quick, this massage remedy induces a heightened mental america and creates profound rest of the body.

- Podikizhi

Podikizhi belongs to the form of Ayurvedic therapies of excessive repute called Sweda. It involves the usage of small linen bags which might be complete of medicated powders prepared from the roots of 12 natural plant life. It is heated and performed anywhere within the frame to result in sweating. Two bundles, containing capsules and the medicated powder, are executed with the useful aid of 2 rubdown therapists to exclusive factors of the frame, simultaneously.

Podikizhi looks after the illnesses because of disrupted Kapha and Vata doshas inclusive of arthritis, rheumatic contamination and spondylosis. Muscular stiffness and sprain additionally can be avoided thru present process this massage treatment as it tones the musculature.

- Elakizhi

Herbal bundles called poultices are prepared with sparkling herbs and leaves as part of this treatment. These bundles are warmed in medicated oils and used for massaging the entire body consisting of the neck, fingers, shoulders and the lower back at the equal time as transferring the man or woman element to aspect. The remedy substantially reduces chronic ache.

- Navrakizhi

Milk and crimson rice are cooked together with natural ayurvedic herbs to make a kheer or pudding. The identical is later amassed in Potalis or boluses and massaged over the pores and skin. It works as an intensely invigorating remedy. It is recommended for people who complain of generalized vulnerable issue and coffee strength. This rubdown is also encouraged for brides-to-be as an herbal frame polish.

- Netra Basti/Netra Tarpanam

We are constantly bombarded with robust optical stimuli due to which our eyes enjoy worn-out and strained, developing poor results on our imaginative and prescient and moreover on the thoughts's interest. Netra Basti can help save you this by using generating a chilled impact on the eyes and the encompassing tissues. The remedy consists of a light facial rub down that emphasizes on the Marma points around the lymph nodes and the eyes. Subsequently, dough jewelry are located round every eye forming a dam. Then, the eyes are bathed in heat ayurvedic Ghee (herbal clarified butter). This nurtures and revitalizes the eyes. Later, eye physical games are done and the Marma elements at the fingers are gently massaged. Thereafter, a Marma detail massage for the face, neck, head and the shoulder completes the enjoy. This rubdown is right for humans laid low with diabetes associated eye troubles and computer imaginative and prescient syndrome.

- Griva Basti / Kati Basti

Griva refers to the neck location, at the identical time as Kati refers to the decrease yet again and hip location. In those localized treatment options, a round-normal dam of wheat flour is sealed throughout the indicated area and a dough ring is full of heat natural oil, which is continuously replenished. Later, the dough ring is eliminated and the region massaged by way of way of manner of emphasizing the Marma elements. The treatment concludes with moderate stretching of the community muscle businesses. The remedy allows to relieve pain in the community regions, especially even as related to degenerative bony modifications.

- Kavialyam

This massage treatment is ready exfoliating the pores and pores and skin with herbs like sesame, ginger, clove, cardamom and first rate powders jumbled in pink rice. It concludes with the software software of an herbal percentage this is produced from licorice at the entire frame. Licorice acts as an anti-tanning agent and allows inside the elimination of pigmentation.

- Sayujyam

This remedy consists of scrubbing the frame with pink rice, tamarind and herbs followed through the usage of a yogurt and tamarind p.C.. Then, the frame is included thru herbal or banana leaves to make a frame wrap. Tamarind includes herbal AHAs that assist in the elimination of tan, on the same time as yogurt permits thru bleaching the skin. The synergistic effect of both makes the pores and pores and skin glowing and colorful.

- Nasyam

In this treatment, therapists rubdown the pinnacle body, from the shoulders to stimulate sweating. A dose of natural medicinal drug is then poured into each nostril. While doing this, the vicinity for the duration of the shoulders, nose and neck is massaged constantly. This treatment is strong in assuaging sinus, chronic colds, headaches, migraines, chest congestion and throat problems. It is likewise diagnosed to soothe and nourish the whole fearful tool.

Chapter 12: Ayurveda and highbrow health

It's normal for any person to sense concerned or disturbing, happy or unhappy, forced or forgetful every now and then. These are the hills and valleys of feelings that every one the human beings experience in their day by day lives. But whilst these feelings or thoughts frequently trouble them and cause disruption in their lives, they'll be laid low with a highbrow infection.

According to the World Health Organization (WHO), more than four hundred million humans across the world are suffering from mental or behavioral troubles. However, figuring out that someone has a highbrow illness and which one it might be, is the first-class undertaking psychiatrists face in recent times due to the reality the signs of maximum of these problems overlap.

Even no matter the fact that the superiority of mental infection is as excessive as one in every five human beings, it no matter the truth that includes a social stigma and discrimination because of which the sufferers and their own family individuals are reluctant to actually get hold of the hassle and are searching for for treatment. Unfortunately, on the same time as mental contamination is left untreated, it may bring about suicide. Ayurveda can provide a holistic treatment for such sufferers via supplying them secure and natural natural medicinal pills.

The facts of highbrow fitness in Ayurvedic treatment

Ayurveda perspectives every person as a very unique mixture of frame, thoughts and spirit, alongside side the psychology and emotions. It consists of rejuvenation, toughness and self-interest treatments the usage of herbs, yoga, weight loss program, breathing wearing sports, meditation, rub down, aromas and mantras.

Ayurveda uses the idea of 3 doshas; vata, pitta and kapha, which while unbalanced, may have an impact on us mentally inflicting disturbed feelings and thoughts. This is normally contemplated at a physical degree additionally and visa versa. Here is a listing of a few intellectual fitness issues which might be not unusual nowadays and the ayurvedic treatment for the same.

Depression

Depression can be defined as a extended us of a of unhappiness or a enjoy of hopelessness, this is frequently followed by using the use of no highs or lows. It represents a mere bland existence that frequently leads to thoughts of suicide. Depression is characterized with the aid of the usage of a problem in doing duties, lack of motivation, reduced urge for meals, quick interest span, crying spells or irregular sleep sample.

Ayurveda believes that the want to arouse the victim's enthusiasm or hobby in lifestyles may be done with the aid of introducing a revel in of taste. Spices like cardamom, ginger and basil are used to open the mind and coronary coronary heart. Calamus teas can be given with honey and ginger. Sages and mints of every type are beneficial. Color therapy is regularly used by ayurvedic specialists to elevate moods in depression patients. The remedy uses heat tones of yellow and gold to arouse a enjoy of positivity inside the mind.

Cutting or causing self-harm

Self-damage involves causing physical harm on one's self this is extreme enough to move away marks that last numerous hours or purpose tissue damage. Cutting is the most common shape of self-harm. Patients can also moreover additionally try burning, biting, hair pulling, pores and skin-deciding on, scratching and head banging due to the fact the technique for inflicting self-damage. Although suicidal emotions may additionally moreover accompany this form of behavior, it does no longer continually mean a severe try to suicide. Most usually, it's miles actually a mechanism for getting over an emotional misery.

Ayurveda makes use of nervine herbs like cayenne, Trikatu, cardamom, calamus and cloves for controlling such behaviors. The nourishing and warming effect of those herbs feed an emotional and sensitive coronary heart. Pippali given with 1/four teaspoon of honey every few hours is likewise precise.

Anxiety Disorders

These encompass panic attacks, positioned up-traumatic strain disease, obsessive-compulsive infection, hypochondria, anger troubles and phobias. These problems are characterised via a effective feeling of panic collectively with the physical signs of fear like trembling, sweating and a racing coronary coronary heart for no obvious purpose the least bit. Ayurveda considers tension as a Vata ailment and recommends Ashwagandha for such patients. It may be given times an afternoon in heat milk. Aromatherapy, the usage of jasmine and rose, is likewise located to be useful in assuaging the tension.

Eating Disorders

There are three forms of ingesting troubles; bulimia nervosa, anorexia nervosa and binge consuming sickness. Each of these has a unique effect on the health of someone. These troubles had been generally related to greater youthful women. However, they may be now acting in younger men as nicely. Anorexia is characterised with the resource of a sudden, significant weight reduction normally because of excessive food plan. Patients see themselves to be overweight, irrespective of their actual weight. People with bulimia nervosa engage in cycles of binging or gorging themselves on large portions of meals after which using laxatives or purging strategies like vomiting to rid the frame of extra strength. It can purpose strain at the bowel muscle groups ensuing in excessive headaches. Repeated vomiting can reason erosion of the tooth of the enamel because of the acid coming from the belly.

Ayurveda recommends those patients to speedy on orange juice and water for the number one three-five days first of all. During this period, the bowels need to be cleansed with a warm water enema as quickly as everyday. After this everyday, they may be capable of adopt an all-fruit weight-reduction plan for the following five days, taking 3 meals an afternoon, comprising of juicy culmination at 5 hourly intervals. Thereafter, they could adopt a food regimen of gently cooked vegetables, buttermilk and juicy stop result for approximately 10 days. Patients can also devour teas of cardamom, smooth ginger or fennel to alter their digestion and prevent vomiting.

Attention-Deficit Hyperactivity Disorder (ADHD)

ADHD is a common behavioral disease affecting school-age youngsters. Children with ADHD are impulsive, hyperactive and function trouble focusing. They can't take a seat down nonetheless, pay attention to information or pay attention.

Ayurveda advises a unique weight-reduction plan for ADHD kids to help accurate the imbalance of doshas within the frame. The healthy dietweight-reduction plan ought to encompass culmination, greens and grains which may be rich in herbal vitamins, enzymes and minerals. Caffeine, sugar, processed meals, MSG and one of a kind sugar substitutes need to be removed from the weight loss plan. Any food containing meals dyes, preservatives or distinctive chemical materials must be averted. Herbal drugs like Brahmi, Basil and Ashwagandha are advocated for boosting the reminiscence and interest span of the sufferers and for controlling their hyperactive and impulsive behavior.

Chapter 13: Pranayam: The Science and Art of Breathing

Breath is Life!

If you have got were given got ever been to a yoga elegance, you should've heard endless praises of deep breathing sports activities. The specific approach of diaphragmatic respiratory engaging the stomach muscle groups and the whole ribcage can assist humans save you numerous disorders and be in the exceptional fitness. It is the reality that the depth and the rhythm of our breath straight away affect the dominion of our body and the mind. According to Ayurveda, breath is a carrier of Prana, the very stress, which gives life to the body. In smooth terms - No breath, no electricity and no lifestyles!

The ancient sages taught us that the "Prana", the crucial deliver of strength circulating within us, may be channeled and cultivated through a spectrum of breathing physical video video games through way of practising pranayam. Pranayam is a focal point-based definitely practice in ayurveda that regulates and controls the breath. It has a mysterious energy to revitalize and soothe a worn-out frame. It can re-energize a wavering mind or a flagging spirit. In the manner, the thoughts is calmed and uplifted.

There are severa Pranayam strategies; but we must pick the right one based totally absolutely at the character needs. If executed nicely, it could offer treasured health benefits. The seven respiratory physical video games in Ayurveda are defined below:

1.   Bhastrika :

Take deep breaths and launch. Fill up your lungs completely at the same time as inhaling and stress the complete breath out. Do it in a rhythm. Imagine that each one the power from the universe is getting into indoors your frame and soul. Feel that each one your pollution and negativity are being expelled out. Practice this for five minutes as soon as each day to live in suitable fitness. Do this instances each day if you are ill.

Bhastrika is useful in treating all forms of pores and skin troubles which include continual problems like leucoderma. People tormented by bizarre discoloration because of burns have moreover benefitted from practicing this pranayam truly.

2.   Kapalbhati

Inhale the air deeply as although taking it into your tummy and breathe out with a jerk. Make positive simplest your belly actions while practicing this and no longer the body. Breathing out need to float the Adam's apple as it pushes thru the throat. You ought to try this for fifteen mins every day, 5 minutes each, three times.

This respiration exercising permits people with most cancers and extraordinary continual conditions. These patients can exercising this for half of-hour each day. It additionally allows people with diabetes. It motives regeneration of the insulin generating beta cells and improves the metabolism of carbohydrates. It additionally improves the fitness of the coronary heart by way of taking off the blocked arteries.

three. Bahya Pranayam

Take deep breaths and launch. Push the stomach in genuinely and keep as you force the breath out. Move your head downwards till the chin touches the better part of the torso. Hold this role for 10-15 seconds after which pass the top up and breathe in. Repeat this for about five-11 instances.

four. Agnisar

Take a deep breath and breathe out. Pull the stomach in even as breathing out. Hold the breath for 15 seconds whilst you flow the stomach inner and out. Then breathe in again. Repeat this three-five instances. This pranayam approach allows humans with digestive troubles like Irritable Bowel Syndrome, gastritis, continual constipation and indigestion.

five. Anulom Bilom

Anulom Bilom is a completely essential pranayam approach. Sit straight away and close to the right nostril alongside side your thumb. Place the index finger on the brow and breathe in deeply via the left nose. Then, near the left nose with the hoop and little fingers joined collectively and breathe out through the proper nostril. Then, take a deep breath through the right nostril, near it with the thumb and breathe out thru the left nostril. This paperwork one cycle of Anulom Bilom. Repeat this cycle for five minutes. This pranayam opens all of the closed channels, recharges the entire frame and re-directs the flow of energy in the frame.

6. Bhramari

Close your ears with the index finger and the center finger. Close the eyes and relaxation the thumb finger at the forehead. Keep the mouth closed. Then, take a deep breath and launch it thru the nostrils with a loud noise from the throat. The noise need to reverbate via the entire frame. Repeat the exercising 5-11 instances. Pranayam will lighten up your mind and body and spark off all of the glands inside the head.

7. Udgeeth

This is a completely exciting pranayam. Take a deep breath. Release the breath through the mouth making the sound "Om". Repeat this 5-

11 times. This brings you closer to the divine element internal you.

Here are a few blessings of Pranayam:

- Breath = Life. Our electricity stages depend on our breath. The fuller you breathe; the more strength your frame and thoughts could have. Taking deeper breaths moreover brings in extra oxygen into the organs and tissues. Consider pranayam as being in an oxygen cafe!

- Deep breaths lessen stress and beautify the digestion. Slow breaths set off the parasympathetic worried system, which gives the body a danger to regenerate, get higher and heal.

- Pranayam enables to strengthen the immune machine and improves the capacity of the frame to fight infections.

- Deep breaths ensure much less inflammation! Most sorts of most cancers arise because of infection. Deep respiratory bodily activities reduce inflammation inside the frame thereby minimizing your hazard of maximum cancers.

• Deep breaths moreover improve one's recognition ranges. It makes you be extra privy to the prevailing moment and helps you to hook up with your instinct. Your body is aware of exactly what and whilst to feed itself to live wholesome, how a brilliant deal to transport and what form of to relaxation. Learning to be aware of that inner voice and expertise it could assist us follow what is extremely good for the body and stay in appropriate fitness.

• Slower breaths additionally make sure higher relationships. Most relationships may be superior if humans are a exceptional deal a good deal much less reactive. If you're capable of step lower lower lower back mentally and expect in advance than speaking, as opposed to saying a few aspect mean; you could contribute plenty to growing a remarkable courting. When you're irritated or annoyed, your breaths are speedy and shortened. When you are calm and cushty, the breaths are sluggish and entire. Pranayam teaches one to control the breath so one can control anger and allows you to have a look at the scenario from a trendy mind-set.

Chapter 14: The blessings of Ayurveda

The recovery device of ayurveda gives severa health advantages. That is the motive humans the world over are turning to this natural treatment for treating their ailments and for preventing diseases. Here are a few blessings of ayurvedic device of medication:

● Ayurvedic drug treatments are organized from natural natural herbs. They do now not contain any chemical substances. Hence, they are unfastened from dangerous aspect consequences. Besides, every herb has specific medicinal houses and a nice flavor and aroma. These herbs act as an super mechanism to result in a balanced synergy most of the frame, mind and spirit and promise to preserve the lifestyles indefinitely. In evaluation to the synthetic capsules, the ones natural drugs are taken into consideration lots more secure.

● Ayurvedic generation does not have a disorder-particular technique. Ayurveda interests at genetically figuring out the trends of the internal as well as out of doors capabilities of a person in place of virtually focusing on curing the sickness. Herbal capsules create an inner concord among unique organs of the frame and additionally some of the body and the encompassing surroundings. These capsules rejuvenate the entire frame tool and now not genuinely cope with a particular ailment.

• The holistic method of ayurvedic herbs aids in proper absorption and digestion. They additionally act as an appetizer. The herbs act as a deliver of easy strength for the thoughts and the soul except appearing rather for proteins, vitamins and vital minerals.

• The recovery value of ayurveda tiers in a huge spectrum and acts as a preventive medicinal drug. It lets in in the rejuvenation of the entire immune device. It complements the strength stages inside the frame and enlightens the soul, mind and the cognitive organs.

• Ayurvedic tablets are particularly useful in treating metabolic troubles without using hormonal dietary dietary supplements. The herbs act at the frame as a whole and enhance the co-ordination amongst diverse hormone-secreting organs to ensure correct balance of the hormones.

• The treatment works at par with the allopathic drugs in terms of remedy and treatment; however the remedy is brought approximately with out causing any horrible results. Ayurveda additionally gives treatment for hard sicknesses like cancer and AIDS.

• Herbal remedies are nutritive and self-contained rendering them non-toxic and nourishing for the frame.

• Ayurveda offers with not genuinely the scientific technology, however also with the social, highbrow, moral and spiritual aspects of the existence of a person.

• Ayurvedic remedy is non-invasive in nature. It can be used as an alternative treatment or along distinct traditional remedy options.

• The natural factors utilized in ayurvedic drug remedies are derived from herbs, vegetation, flowers, end result, and so on. Making the treatment and the whole enjoy towards the person.

• The useful impact of ayurvedic remedy lasts for an extended period in assessment to the allopathic pills whose motion lasts handiest for a specific length. The stop result of herbal remedy is generally eternal and allows someone keep away from recurrence of the infection.

• Ayurvedic drug remedies can be used in spite of the useful resource of healthy people as they will be restorative in nature and assist in improving intellectual functionality and nourishment of the frame.

• Ayurvedic remedy and natural drug remedies are a good deal inexpensive than different systems of medicine.

• Ayurveda recommends effects to be had kitchen herbs and spices for minor illnesses. These drug remedies can also take delivery of to youngsters and aged patients with out the concern of unfavorable reaction.

• Dubbed due to the fact the "era of existence" or the "know-how of lifestyles," Ayurveda can assist human beings beautify the overall amazing in their lifestyles.

- A multitude of herbs in ayurveda are blended collectively to fight and prevent immune issues. These combos are believed to assist help the frame's protection mechanisms simply so the illnesses have lots less risk of settling in.

The philosophy of ayurveda consists of a series of conceptual structures which are characterised via health and ailment, balance and disease. Health/illness is a give up end result of interconnectedness or the dearth of it amongst the whole thing that takes place in the bodily, highbrow, emotional and spiritual being. To continue to be healthful, there need to be a concord between the thoughts, feelings and physical movements. Ayurvedic medicinal drugs collectively with yoga, meditation, massage remedy plans and respiratory sports help humans gain this harmony and maintain remaining health. After an ayurvedic remedy, a person exhibits an ordinary improvement of their physical, highbrow and mental state.

Chapter 15: image-placeholder

The word Ayurveda originated from the historical Indian Sanskrit language. Ayu manner "life," and Veda way "knowledge." So Ayurveda manner "know-how of life." The exercising originated in India greater than 6,000 years ago. Ayurveda is a herbal and holistic approach to mental and physical fitness. Modern medicinal drug focuses on remedying health issues.

In assessment, Ayurveda specializes in preventing them. Ayurveda takes a holistic approach to treating and preventing illnesses. Ayurveda advocates that after a person is mentally and physically in shape, they're able to hold themselves in a totally great nation of thoughts and electricity and obtain their existence desires. Ayurveda is often known as the "Mother of all Healing" due to its holistic nature of restoration.

Many enlightened sages spend limitless years running towards deep meditation to accumulate Ayurvedic know-how. Then passes in this recognize-the way to their disciples. The exercising began out as an oral lifestyle and unfold inside the path of the Indian subcontract through phrase of mouth. Around 2,500 years inside the past, Ayurvedic teachings had been recorded in writing. The Charaka Samhita – the primary Ayurvedic scripture, modified into written. The Sushruta Samhita and Ashtanga Hridayam are the possibilitymanuscripts that exist in recent times. These three manuscripts keep all of the philosophies, requirements, and practices of Ayurveda.

Ayurveda sees a person as an covered being: mind, body, and spirit. It is a preventive clinical tool that encourages chronic health and sturdiness. Ayurveda is an all-inclusive clinical device that consists of: stylish treatment, geriatrics, ear/nose/throat, ophthalmology, obstetrics, gynecology, pediatrics, psychotherapy, and surgical treatment. Ayurveda considers all factors of your lifestyles and deploys various healing strategies to treat, heal, and rejuvenate your health.

Energy is in us and all spherical us. Energy influences all residing matters. The ayurvedic workout believes that every dwelling problem contains a balance of 5 factors: earth, air, fireside, water, and ether (space). These 5 factors play critical roles in balancing our bodily and nonphysical our our our bodies. They are active forces that have an impact on the whole lot we do every day, together with our notion styles, environment, food, digestion, the form of sleep we've got, the way we flow into our our our bodies, and so forth. Once you start to recognize and sense the interactions of these diffused energies in your frame and your lifestyles, you can start to stability yourself.

image-placeholder

The Three Doshas - Finding your balance

Ayurveda workout tells us that the 5 energetic factors make up the 3 doshas: Vata, Pitta, and Kapha. These factors are present in our our our bodies, and additionally they may be found inside the changing seasons, the sports we do, the food we devour, the surroundings we live in, and the relationships we have were given.

The 3 doshas are used to define the lively stability of our being. The precise dosha stability internal every mother and father is decided at idea and stays the same in the course of our lives. However, internal and out of doors elements can unbalance it. Our doshic stability impacts our emotional and highbrow inclinations, likes and dislikes, physical tendencies, tendencies within the route of specific behavior, and vulnerability to illness. Once you start to apprehend that the active factors interior your body and in nature – are composed of these three doshas, you have got were given started out to recognize the idea of Ayurveda.

image-placeholder

Vata

•Governs: All physical motion

•Elements: air and ether (area)

•Elemental functions: Mobile, quick, moderate, dry, bloodless, abnormal, and difficult

•Seasons: Late fall (autumn) and early wintry weather

•Body parts: Colon, small intestine, and huge gut

•Physical abilities: Individuals with a Vata nature predominate the air detail. This makes Vatas thin, with mild and wiry structure, prolonged angular abilities, and small dark eyes which is probably normally brown.

Vata's personalities resemble the characteristics of air and place. This is why their body sorts have a tendency to be tall, thin, and lanky. Their mind and sports activities are mild, short, and rapidly converting. Vata energy is located inside the mind, pores and skin, joints, bones, colon, nerves, muscle groups, legs, and toes. Vata governs the motion of your frame, so it's far crucial to hold it in balance. Processes like thoughts, mobility, muscle tension, blinking, respiratory, heartbeat, circulate, and waste elimination – all are managed via Vata.

When your Vata is in concord

You will revel in brilliant vibrancy, creativity, and strength with heightened memory, reasoning, senses, and not unusual sense. You can be able to digest meals properly and take away waste with out trouble. Vata's persona is; clearly happy, excitable, and modern-day. They like hot weather and warmth food. However, they will be predisposed to be forgetful. They are typically very social and notable communicators. Vatas like to have fun and are short to chortle at a celebration. They do not like physical games and might adjust to closing-minute changes in plans. This is why Vatas ought to try to hold everyday schedules, behavior, and practices to keep themselves in balance.

Moderate excessive sports activities are best for Vata doshas due to the truth they will hold them engaged without overwhelming them. Competitive, strenuous, difficult, or frenetic exercising routines can throw them out of balance. Meditative sports together with qigong, tai chi, strolling, Pilates, yoga, or swimming supplement their workouts properly.

The downside of Vata

They get overexerted and overworked, at the same time as confronted with a busy way of existence, Vatas fast grow to be imbalanced and overstimulated. They can lack willpower and become bored short. If you're Vata inclined, then those signs and symptoms and signs and symptoms and signs and symptoms will can help you understand that you are out of stability:

•Cold palms and feet

•Headaches, earaches, coughs, sore throat

•Body aches or fatigue

•Gas, constipation, bloating, or diarrhea

•Pain in the decrease decrease once more or stomach

•Dry or brittle hair

•Skin problems along side roughness, dryness, and breakouts

•Distracting mind, a racing mind

•Difficulty with drowsing

•Stress, tension, worry, worry

•Bringing decrease lower back stability thru food

When Vatas want to grow to be cool and calm, they need warmer, heavier, moister, or oiler meals which might be candy, sour, or salty in flavor (which includes roasted greens, heat milk, thick stews, warm cereals, or nuts). They must keep away from meals which may be raw, bitter, smelly, crunchy, crispy, dry, cold, similarly to cold or raw vegetables. They have to moreover keep away from carbonated beverages collectively with sodas and seltzers.

Foods that soothe an imbalance and help Vata :

•Eggs, wild-caught seafood, natural bird or turkey, pork

•Dairy, which consist of warmth milk (boiled in keeping with ayurvedic commands) and yogurt

•Wheat and rice. (Reduce quantities of millet, buckwheat, oats, and rye)

•Nuts of any type

•Oils of a wide variety

•Mung dahl, tofu/soy, and unique small beans. (Lower quantities of gasoline-generating beans alongside side artisan, white, red, kidney, and black)

•All kinds of sweeteners, which includes sugar, fruit extracts, agave, and honey carefully

•Fruits (eaten alone if feasible) that have a tendency to be candy, sour, or heavy (melons, candy berries, papaya, mango, pineapples, bananas, cherries, avocado, peaches) limit intake of dry, dried, and mild types, collectively with pomegranates, cranberries, citrus, pears, and apples.

•Organic cooked greens: beets, carrots, and asparagus. When cooked with Vata-boosting spices (fairly): broccoli, cauliflower, celery, potatoes, and leafy vegetables. Avoid cabbage and sprouts.

•Most warming spices and sparkling herbs (revel in pepper cautiously). Especially useful are mustard seed, cloves, cumin, salt, cinnamon, ginger, and cardamom.

•Activities that resource Vata

•Besides weight-reduction plan, you may do various things to preserve your Vata energies balanced

•Vata is vulnerable to colds, so keep on with warmness temperatures. Stay warm temperature whilst temperatures drop.

•Eat warm temperature factors. (Limit raw and chilled meals)

•Choose comfort foods which might be oily, heavy, and warmth (which consist of roasts, casseroles, and stews).

•Practice outstanding sleep behavior. Go to mattress early and awaken early.

•Massage your body with sesame oil.

•Avoid things that stimulate you.

•Maintain a day by day ordinary to keep away from tension, stress, and fear

•Drink heat spiced milk earlier than bed to encourage sleep

•Gym often

•Enjoy one-of-a-type sports and pursuits that keep your thoughts active.

image-placeholder

Kapha

•Governs: The form of the body and the formation of all seven tissues: Bones, marrow, fat, muscle, blood, nutritive fluid, and reproductive tissues

•Elements: Water and earth

•Elemental characteristics: Static, dense, robust, heavy, oily, moist, cool

•Seasons: Late wintry climate and early spring

•Body additives: Throat, lungs, nostrils, sinuses, and lungs

•Physical skills: Kapha individuals have a predominance of water elements. Their thick, cool, gentle, and wet pores and pores and skin reflects this element. Kaphas normally tend to have a huge frame, stocky construct, a properly-advanced chest, nicely-lubricated joints, and a well-proportioned and sturdy frame. Kaphas have problem losing weight, simply so they have a tendency to be obese.

Kapha human beings mirror the features of water and earth. Kapha frame sorts have a tendency to be obese, heavier, and extra prominent. Their movements and thoughts are sluggish, slower, and vulnerable to despair. Kapha energy is located in the chest, ligaments, tendons, throat and lungs, fatty tissues, and connective tissues.

When Kapha is in harmony, they may experience feelings of pleasure, happiness, love, and forgiveness. They can be generous, affectionate, comfortable, and easygoing. With a low, mild voice, large, inviting eyes, and cushty actions, kaphas come upon as calm, tranquil, and serene.

These skills regularly located them in apprehend or management roles in their social circles, companies, and companies. Dependable or perhaps-keeled, you can assume them for the duration of a excessive-stress, worrying scenario. Kaphas additionally pride themselves on being reliable, devoted, strong, reliable, and understanding. Physically they will be large, heavier, sturdier, and extra grounded than special doshas. When they will be out of balance, they have a propensity to be extra sluggish. Kaphas are not quick learners, but they might go through in mind records higher than others.

To keep away from weight advantage, kaphas must workout slight-intensity aerobic sports activities. Unlike vatas, kaphas need to interact in strenuous sporting occasions or sports activities to preserve themselves inspired and stimulated. They are well at soccer, basketball, and marathon walking. Practicing meditative activities collectively with qigong, walking, Pilates, yoga, and tai chi is proper for them.

Kaphas can address strain well, and that they have got a snug demeanor. They have exceptional health with powerful immune structures. When out of balance, kaphas can become lazy, addictive, overly linked, touchy, and possessive. If you are Kapha, then those are the signs and symptoms and signs and symptoms so you can allow you to comprehend that you are out of stability:

- Excessive dozing or dozing

- Addictions

- Oversensitivity

- Lifeless outlook on life

- Dry pores and pores and skin or hair

- Difficult or toxic relationships

- Resistance to change

- Feelings of possessiveness

- Homebody tendencies

- Difficulty with social engagements

- Lacking desire for physical or intellectual stimulation

- Bad TV behavior

- Laziness, no exercising

- Emotional ingesting, bingeing

- Problems with overeating

- Asthma, hypersensitive reactions, headaches, sinus troubles, congestion, flu, colds

•Cellulite

•Excess weight

•Judgment, jealousy, envy, lack of confidence

Bring lower returned stability through ingredients

When kaphas need motivation, delight, and perception, they have to opt for warming, spicy, dry, or moderate foods that deliver them a lift of strength. Think zesty citrus, spiced teas, or substances with pepper, garlic, or ginger. They need to avoid watery, sweet, cold, sour, and heavy meals.

If you feel imbalanced, then use the ones food to hold your energies balanced:

•Buckwheat, millet, barley, and rye over wheat, rice, and oats

•All varieties of beans, besides soybeans

•Ginger tea

•Limited quantity of oil. Choose mustard oil, almond oil, ghee, and olive oil

•A small wide kind of nuts and seeds. Sunflower and pumpkin seeds cautiously

•All sorts of spices. Opt for easy cinnamon, cumin, chilies, black pepper, and ginger. Avoid salt.

•All forms of natural vegetables. Avoid greens which can be greater sugary, starchier, and wet, like tomatoes, corn, squash, zucchini, and candy potatoes.

•Endive

•Eat common smaller meals. Eat a larger meal at lunchtime and eat little or no at dinner. Avoid consuming some thing three hours earlier than sleep.

•Choose lighter give up end result along side apricots, pomegranates, cranberries, pears, and apples. Avoid heavier options like figs, dates, melons, bananas, stone fruits, and tropical surrender result.

•More uncooked meals than cooked

•Consume astringent, bitter, and smelly additives. Avoid buttery, sugary, or oily options.

•Take uncooked honey in constrained quantities. Avoid other varieties of sweeteners.

•Spicy, warm, stimulating substances, flavors, or cuisines

•Warm food, coffees, and teas. Avoid cold food and drink

•Citrus flavors like lemon or lime

Activities that help Kapha

Besides those components, you may integrate various things into your life to keep Kapha energies in balance:

•New or unique exercises or sports which consist of a exchange in hobbies, a in addition gym class, or a new course to paintings

•Social sports

•Experiences that enlarge, circulate, or have interaction your frame, thoughts, or spirit in a special way

•Stimulating sports that need frenetic movements or short wondering

•Avoid oily, sugary, or processed additives

•Avoid immoderate enjoyment, relaxation, or indulgence.

•Early to mattress and early to upward thrust. Avoid naps

•Stay decided to hold your every day ordinary

•Spend time in heat environments together with seashores or saunas

•Use rejuvenating important oils consisting of eucalyptus to maintain you energized

•Avoid lethargy. Stretch, walk, or motorcycle after food

•Avoid emotional consuming by using way of using distracting your self. Engage in an interest which you love; walk, or speak to a pal

•Give your self a dry self-massage in the morning and at night time time. This will boom movement and power stages.

•Focus on competitive, frenetic, uplifting, or tough sports, like aerobics, cycling, kickboxing, walking, or dancing.

•Choose fabrics with interesting styles or brilliant colorations.

image-placeholder

Pitta

•Governs: The transformation of food and thoughts

•Elements: Fire and water

•Elemental capabilities: Smooth, clean, sharp/precise, cell, liquid, slight, oily, heat

•Seasons: Summer

•Body additives: Pancreas, duodenum, stomach, gallbladder, spleen, liver

•Physical capabilities: Pitta people have a predominance of the fire element. Pittas generally tend to have a medium-sized construct and moderate muscle tone. Their pores and pores and skin is typically wet, slight, reddish, warm, and sincere, with an inclination inside the path of rashes and zits. Their eyes are medium-sized and moderate in coloration with slight-colored hair.

•Sensitivities: Sensitive to humidity and heat. Burn rapid inside the solar

Pitta human beings resemble the capabilities of water and fire. Pitta dosha is related to exchange and transformation, so they're usually taken into consideration agile and extra flexible (each in mind and body). Pittas are a median construct, usually generally tend to have warmth or oily pores and skin, strong muscle, and feature plenty of body warmness. Pitta character's mind and moves are expressive, loud, passionate, extreme, and dominating.

Pitta electricity is placed within the pancreas, small intestine, blood, eyes, liver, spleen, belly, and sweat within the frame. When careworn, they typically will be inclined to overheat each mentally and bodily. Their acidic, acerbic, fluid, aggressive, sharp, and hot features cause them to competitive.

When pitta is in concord

They will experience strength, intelligence, attention, self guarantee, and contentment. Strong desires and impulses are characteristics of a pitta person. They are excellent, insightful, and extroverted. Individuals need to be the pitta electricity as it's effective, honestly satisfied, radiant, courageous, and mentally astute. Pittas are rather aggressive, targeted, ambitious, decisive, and a achievement. You will regularly find pitta people at sporting activities. The rebellious and active nature of pittas generally makes them a hit. Characteristics of pittas frequently push them into management roles in politics, company, or social networks.

Pitta humans are self-motivating and do not need greater incentives to participate in competitive or strenuous exercising exercises or sports activities activities sports sports activities sports. They want to be careful about not turning into overly competitive or severe. They want to learn how to revel in subjects greater in preference to commonly focusing on triumphing. Pitta humans have to balance their normal with conscious activities like swimming, qigong, tai chi, strolling, pilates, and yoga.

Here are the signs of unbalanced pitta

•Ulcers

•Signs of suppressed feelings

•Irritability, anger, rage, or judgmental thoughts

•Outbursts, mood tantrums

•Irritation with extraordinary people, each at home and art work

•Skin troubles like zits, pores and pores and skin most cancers, boils, sunburn, bruises, eczema, and rashes

•Thinning hair or baldness

•Overthinking approximately money

•Attention-trying to find inclinations

•Narcissistic

•Addictions like alcohol, caffeine, or nicotine.

•A competitive streak on overdrive

•Mood swings

•Overheating, more sweat

- Bitterness

- Harsh reviews about others

- Inflammation that motives contamination, fever, or sickness

- Acid stomach or heartburn

- Fatigue or insomnia

- Extreme perfectionism

Bringing decrease again balance through foods

Pitta human beings need calming, cooling food to balance their fiery nature. They have to reputation on consuming juicy and candy food. They must avoid acidic, warmth, oily, salty, highly spiced, or sour options.

If you are experiencing imbalance, then use the ones components to balance yourself:

- Eat pomegranate, coconut, dates, lychee, grapes, melons, mango, and apples. Avoid rhubarb, plums, tropical end result, citrus, cherries, berries, and apricots

- All sorts of beans besides for lentils

•Parsnip, celery, zucchini, squash, potatoes, mushrooms, peas, lettuce, celery, asparagus, broccoli, cauliflower, cucumber, Brussels sprouts, and bell peppers. Limit eggplant, avocados, tomatoes, turnip, spinach, radish, pickled veggies, chilies, carrots, and beets.

•Consume ghee, unsalted butter, buttermilk, sweet lassi, and smooth cheese. Limit sour or heavier dairy merchandise like sour cream, tough cheese, sour buttermilk, ice cream, and yogurt.

•Like wheat, oats, rice, and barley, avoid corn, rye, or buckwheat.

•Herbs and spices with cooling and calming houses embody cumin, fennel, dill, coriander, cardamom, rose, mint, lemon-grass, and turmeric. Limit heat generators like chilies, nutmeg, ginger, garlic, sage, cayenne, onion, mustard seed, cinnamon, caraway, bay leaves, and basil.

•Leafy greens like endive, dandelions, arugula, and kale

•Coconut oils, soy, and sunflower oils are higher for this frame type. Use almond, peanut, sesame, corn, and olive oils moderately

•Opt for pumpkin and sunflower seeds. Reduce consumption of all nuts besides coconut. Limit sesame seeds.

•Chilled water, milk, coconut milk, and funky drinks like fruit and vegetable juices are pleasant. Limit heat beverages like tea and espresso. Also, restriction carbonated beverages and alcohol.

•Opt for natural sweeteners like honey, sugar, agave, or fruit nectars. Avoid artificial sweeteners.

Activities that help pitta

Besides weight-reduction plan, proper right here are some sports activities activities to help you keep your pitta energies balanced:

•Spending time in nature

•Spending time with own family and friends in cushty environments, at the side of taking a yoga class together or taking a stroll after dinner

•Gentle physical wearing activities on the aspect of stretching, yoga, strolling, qigong, tai chi, and swimming

•Eating meals at regular durations

•Taking shorter breaks and meditating

•Staying in a moist or cool environment. Avoid warmth, solar, or heat weather.

•Avoiding smoking and alcohol

•If you sense stressed, then unfold 1 tsp. Rose petal jam on toast or crackers and enjoy

•Focus on artwork-existence balance. Avoid overworking

•Limit rather spiced, pickled, and fried meals

•Do nonprofit or charity art work that cultivates kindness, generosity, honesty, staying power, and sharing. Give significance to ethics over competition, aggression, and fulfillment.

•Practice meditation

•Therapy or anger control instructions

•Massage coconut oil on any a part of the frame this is stressful, especially the scalp and ft

•Start your day with ½ cup apple or pomegranate juice combined with ½ cup aloe vera juice. Avoid consuming tea or coffee.

•Induce sleep by taking a cool tub or bathe earlier than going to bed

•After a tough day, stroll within the night time time to lighten up your self

•Relax earlier than mattress with the aid of heading off exercising and electronics

Pitta dosha power spikes among 10 AM and a couple of PM. So eat lunches that consist of cooling meals. Eating the wrong sorts of lunches will motive you to crave meals (chilies, garlic, onions, and one of a kind warming spices and herbs) that make you unbalanced.

image-placeholder

The 6 tastes

Depending for your dosha kind, the ayurvedic diet plan includes six one-of-a-type tastes that actively effect your mind and frame:

•Astringent

•Bitter

•Pungent

•Salty

•Sour

•Sweet

An important and unique detail of Ayurveda "tastes" play in identifying what food to consume.

Each "flavor" is described in terms of the identical elements and capabilities of the doshas and the natural elements (which embody drying, heating, cooling). Because of its functions, every taste will assist stability specific doshas and have an effect on the digestive hearth in any other case.

The following statistics approximately "tastes" affords hints to help you recognize the rate of "tastes" and their traits. You are a unique being, and your wishes shift with time, seasons, and adjustments for your lifestyles.

image-placeholder

image-placeholder

Each taste has multiple impact at the frame and mind. "Tastes" are more fundamental in sweet, sour, and astringent have a cooling effect. "Tastes" dominant in pungent, salty, and bitter have a heating impact.

Examples of ingredients and their tastes

Ayurveda has positioned and documented the developments of the tastes, and the categorizations assist pick out what is top notch for you. You won't be used to spotting the "tastes" in the food you devour because of the truth such treatment of "taste" is not typically considered within the Western view of a healthful food plan.

Because of its tendencies, every flavor has a one-of-a-kind impact to your frame and mind. The simplest manner to recollect the effects is to take into account traits. For example, while you are strolling warm, pick tastes which is probably cooling. If you feel slow and torpid, select out "tastes" associated with fireside to function some kick and stimulate strength on your device.

Tastes for Vata

Remember, the traits associated with Vata are moderate, cold, dry, and cellular. So, you need to ground vata's energy and balance it with these trends: heavy, moist, and heat. The extraordinary tastes for Vata are salty, sweet, and bitter.

•Sweet to ground Vata: Sweet taste is crafted from earth and water factors. The candy flavor has wet and heavy trends, each quick-time period and lengthy-time period. These traits are wonderful for balancing Vata's slight, cellular and dry attributes. Sweet has a slightly cooling impact on the digestive device, but without a doubt enough to provide you a feel of feeling complete or glad.

•Sour's warming and heavy assist: Sour's factors are earth and fireplace, which means that that sour is grounding and healing, with some moisture. The heating outstanding of

136

bitter allows kindle the digestive hearth, making the flavor very supportive for Vata. The warming and grounding results live with the frame beyond the approach of digestion, furthermore very balancing for Vata.

•Salty advantages for Vata: The salty flavor includes hearth and water. Its initial effects at the tool are heating and moistening, which help to balance vata's cool and dry features. The fiery element of the salty taste permits digestion, which can be very supportive for Vata kinds whose appetites may be variable and whose coolness and dryness have an effect at the digestive hearth.

These trends have an effect on the mind, no longer just the frame. So, for example, the grounding awesome of bitter will create emotions of balance and aid, counteracting vata's tendency inside the route of tension and worry.

Chapter 16:image-placeholder

According to Ayurveda, the fitness of the mind and the intestine's fitness are related. Modern era additionally famous that the kingdom of your digestion impacts your mind. According to Scientific American, ninety five% of your serotonin is decided to your bowels. This is why the intestine is regularly known as the second mind. Your intestine is complete of useful micro organism. Your gut, or the "2d brain," carries a hundred million neurons. This microbiome is important in your not unusual health. It works cautiously at the side of your frame's immune tool and weight law. The microbiome controls nutrient absorption, blood glucose, insulin sensitivity, and the manufacturing of severa neurochemicals and neurohormones.

More and additional research are linking the brain and gut health. Poor digestion can motive many intestine troubles, which encompass acidity, GERD, bloating, and diarrhea. When your gut malfunctions, your thoughts gets affected. Here are Ayurvedic strategies for a wholesome gut and maximum green thoughts fitness:

Ayurvedic gadget for intestine health

The following are the subjects you may do to improve your intestine fitness and ignite digestive fireside:

Drink heat water: Drinking warmth water in some unspecified time in the future of the day will stimulate digestion, enhance metabolism, and clean out ama.

Avoid cold drinks: Avoid them, particularly inside the route of your mealtime. Drinking cold drinks at some point of your mealtime diminishes your digestive hearth.

Sit and loosen up even as ingesting: According to Ayurveda, you need to take a seat down down down and lighten up throughout mealtime, take a look at your food and smell it. This will reason saliva manufacturing in your mouth, crucial for digestion. Slowing down and taking slight breaths earlier than food moreover permits your frame input relaxation and digest mode. A calm and comfortable body is essential for digestion.

Chew your food: Chew your food nicely because of the truth it is critical for digestion.

Chewing produces saliva, it's vital for proper digestion. Additionally, chewing slowly offers your intestine time to ship your thoughts a signal that you are full so that you can avoid overeating. Rushing subsequently of consuming will result in overeating.

Eat your largest meal at some point of lunchtime: According to Ayurveda, our digestive fireside is most effective at noon. So you want to eat your biggest meal at midday. This dependancy may even deliver your frame sufficient time to digest your meals earlier than snoozing.

Eat great at the same time as you're hungry: Do now not consume due to the truth it is mealtime. Check to appearance in case you are feeling hungry. If you are not hungry, then take away ingesting. Eating whilst you revel in complete will overload your digestive machine—workout aware consuming.

Five spices: Take the ones five spices (ginger, cardamom, cumin, coriander, and fennel) for maximum ideal digestion. Studies show that those spices help the body produce its digestive enzymes and bile.

Use ghee: Ghee is a have to for Ayurveda cooking. An component in ghee helps you avoid leaky gut syndrome. Leaky intestine syndrome can cause pretty some health problems. Ghee furthermore lubricants your digestive device, so subjects run without problem.

Follow suitable meals combination: Ayurveda recommends proper food combination. Combining meals incorrectly will lessen your Agni or digestive fireplace. This can reason gasoline, bloating, indigestion, and poisonous accumulation. One instance is combining fruit collectively with melon with a few other meals. Fruit is digested fast in advance than specific gradual-digesting food, which can purpose fermentation and bloating. Avoid meals combinations, together with bananas and milk, beans with cheese, and uncooked and cooked components.

Include all six tastes: You need to embody all six tastes (astringent, bitter, stinky, sour, salty, and sweet) for a balanced weight loss plan. Including all six tastes will ensure that you get all the crucial meals agencies and vitamins. It might also make you greater glad and assist you avoid snacking.

Walk after ingesting: According to Ayurveda, you need to stroll for 15 mins after every meal to assist useful useful resource digestion. Studies show that strolling after each meal permits with digestion and balances blood sugar degrees.

Get enough sleep: You want to get sufficient sleep to preserve perfect intestine fitness. Your frame enters into the relaxation and digest country at the same time as you sleep. This offers your body the hazard to digest the whole lot and gives your concerned machine time to recharge for the next day. Preferably, you want to sleep in your left aspect. This allows with proper bowel motion.

image-placeholder

Ayurvedic answers for commonplace stomach issues

1. Constipation: You need to devour a drink made with hot water, salt, and ghee to triumph over this problem. Salt removes bacteria, and ghee lets in lubricate the inner

of the intestines. Also, ingesting a ripe bananahours after dinner and ingesting a tumbler of hot water or heat milk help stop constipation.

Consuming a tbsp. Of (immoderate pleasant, food-grade) castor oil at bedtime moreover permits. However, keep away from this oil in case you are pregnant.

2. Bloated: Mix ginger or fennel seeds in a tumbler of heat water and drink to remedy this hassle. If you do not want to drink whatever, chunk fennel seeds after your food. This aids inside the digestion manner and diminishes gasoline and bloating.

three. Acid reflux: If you have got this problem, then bite clove, holy basil, or fennel seeds. You can mix buttermilk and coconut water and drink it. According to Ayurveda, buttermilk aids digestion soothes the belly and decreases acid reflux disease sickness.

4. Diarrhea: Calabash or bottle gourd is awesome for diarrhea. You can prepare dinner dinner dinner severa dishes with it (which consist of curry, stew, or soup). Avoid

dehydration if you have diarrhea. Drink lots of fluids. Ideally, you ought to drink water, however you may additionally attempt fruit juice, specifically pomegranate, apple juice, or ginger tea. Drinking buttermilk additionally permits.

five. Indigestion: If your belly is upset, undergo in thoughts what you have got eaten over the past 48 hours, and consume some component to counterbalance it. Avoid uncooked veggies, big grains, and dairy that is difficult to digest—Cook veggies with spices that beneficial useful resource in digestion like black pepper, cinnamon, and ginger. Eating soups help in the path of this time. Drinking juices moreover help.

Mix ¼ tsp. Of garlic paste in a glass of buttermilk and drink. Or you may take same portions of honey and onion juice. If you have got got heartburn, acid reflux disease sickness, or infection in your digestive tract, onion and garlic can also worsen it in addition.

Good eating behavior, consistent with Ayurveda

•Incorporate spices like asafetida, coriander, fennel seeds, cumin, and turmeric into your diet plan

•Drink cumin or ginger tea as soon as an afternoon

•Avoid ice-cold food or liquids

•Do no longer drink ice water

•Avoid snacks

•Take small sips of warmth water during your food

•Avoid contradicting meals combinations

Ayurvedic treatments for constipation

Common reasons of constipation

•Parasites

•Imbalance of gut flora

•Congestion within the colon or obstruction due to pollution

•Travel

•Suppression of herbal urges

•High stress

- Irregular sleep habitual

- Lack of sleep or insomnia

- Irregular meal schedule

- Lack of a regular every day recurring

- Excessive fear and worry

- Anxiety

- Dehydration

- Leftovers or stale meals

- Intake of allergenic or insupportable meals (at the side of eggs, nuts, soy, dairy, gluten, and wheat)

- Regular consumption of incorrect food

- Vata-Provoking manner of existence

- Poor nutritional conduct

- Vata-provoking food plan

Ayurvedic remedies for constipation

1. Eating a strict Vata-lowering weight loss program: Eating a wholesome however Vata-horrifying eating regimen (together with dried culmination, raw vegetables, salads, and so

on.) can cause constipation. You want to recognition on consuming a Vata-pacifying weight loss plan. Here are some pointers:

• Eat easy, smooth-to-digest food which include crock-pot, stews, broths, steamed greens, white quinoa, basmati rice, dal, kitchari, soup, and so forth.

• Choose properly-spiced, warmness, and tender components.

• Avoid uncooked, hard, cold, dry food and drinks (which embody granola bars, protein bars, dry cereal, toast, crackers, natural juice, bloodless smoothies, raw greens, and many others.)

• Limit heavy, difficult-to-digest factors which includes beans (except for red lentils and mung beans), meat, and dairy

• Maintain a consistent consuming time desk. For instance, breakfast at 6 – 7 AM, Lunch at eleven – 1 PM, Dinner at 5 – 7 PM.

• Follow the right food combos.

2. Follow a Vata-balancing manner of existence: Follow Vata-lowering life-style

practices to address Vata imbalance. This will address constipation and assist with unique Vata imbalance troubles together with pressured mind, anxiety, and sleep troubles. Here are a few Vata-decreasing steps that you can take

•Maintain a Vata-precise sleep time desk. For instance, go to bed at 9 – 10 PM. Wake up at 6 – 7 AM.

•Maintain a consistent every day routine

•Practice deep belly respiratory 3 times each day

•Practice restorative yoga severa times every week

•Take a heat ginger bathtub several instances every week

•Before mattress, use Vata oil to massage your body. Do this numerous times every week.

3. Avoid bloodless or iced water and drink heat water: Drink heat water after waking up and constantly amongst food. Drink a complete of 8 to 10 cups of warm water. This

will maintain you hydrated and keep away from constipation. Drinking warm water opens the critical channels within the frame, receives rid of the obstruction, flush out the GI tract, and useful resource in wholesome removal.

Directions: Start your day via ingesting sixteen ozof warm water. Then drink sixteen oz. Of warm temperature water among every meal. Do no longer drink some aspect in the direction of your meals or after a meal.

4. Consume this smoothie made with papaya each morning: This recipe is made with warming spices warmth water and includes substances that sell removal. Papaya can be very powerful for treating constipation. Recipe:

•1 tsp. Honey

•1 tsp. Coconut oil

•¼ tsp. Cinnamon

•1/8 tsp. Cardamom

•Fresh ginger, thinly sliced

•½ cup heat water

•½ of a medium papaya

Method: Blend the whole thing in a blender for 2 minutes. Drink this after you've got consumed 16 ouncesof warm water in the morning. Avoid consuming whatever for 1/2-hour.

five. 1 tsp. Soaked chia seeds: When because it want to be taken, chia seeds can lubricate the colon and cope with constipation. Soak 1 tsp. Chia seeds in water and take it in the morning. This will beneficial useful resource in healthful elimination.

Method: Soak 1 tsp. Of chia seeds in 1 cup of water in a single day. Then take it after you have ate up sixteen oz.Of warm water inside the morning.

6. Warm milk, honey, ghee, and haritaki: Mix those components and make a drink. Then drink it in advance than bed. Haritaki can lessen Vata and is mainly powerful toward constipation.

Method: In a pan, warm temperature ½ cup of milk, however do now not boil it. Then get rid of from the warmth. Add 1 tsp. Ghee and 1 tsp. Haritaki. Mix well and cool barely (108 ranges or much less). Then stir in 1 tsp. Honey. Drink this 15 mins in advance than bed.

7. 1 tsp. Triphala Churna: Take 1 tsp. Triphala churna each night time before mattress. Triphala Churna (Churna manner powdered) is made with the aggregate of 3 forestall end result: Haritaki, Bibhitaki, and Amalaki. These 3 dried stop result are blended and then crushed to make a powder. This is robust Ayurvedic medicinal drug. It enables deal with severa sicknesses and signs and symptoms, which includes irritation and constipation.

Method: In 1 cup of warmth water, steep 1 tsp. Of Triphala Churna for five minutes. Drink it 15 to half of-hour earlier than mattress.

8. 1 spoonful of Vata honey infusion: Before every meal, take a spoonful of Vata honey infusion to cope with constipation. Vata honey is a digestive beneficial aid that enables with severa digestive problems, along

with bloating, gas, and constipation. Take this treatment in advance than every meal to ignite your digestive fireside, digest and assimilate food well and promote wholesome elimination.

Method: Consume 1 tsp. Of Vata honey infusion earlier than each meal. Then drink a chunk of heat water. You want to try this each day to address constipation.

9. Vata honey and Triphala Churna: Take the onesdevices earlier than bed every night time time. If you have got a immoderate constipation problem, take thoseremedies collectively in advance than mattress each night time time time. Vata honey and Triphala Churna help reduce Vata, help to create balance in the GI tract, and cope with constipation.

Method: Mix 1 tsp. Triphala Churna and 1 tbsp. Vata honey to make a soupy paste. Take this each night time time earlier than bed, then drink ½ cup of warmth water. If you've got were given have been given severe constipation, then repeat inside the morning.

10. Weekly Dashamul Tea Basti: This remedy is specially powerful toward constipation and Vata imbalance.

Method: Perform the Dashamula tea Basti, on an empty belly first detail within the morning or in advance than bed. Repeat the technique numerous instances each week until your constipation has dwindled.

eleven. Take ginger tea blended with castor oil: You need to apply terrific, natural, food-grade castor oil for this recipe. Castor oil is a powerful treatment to address constipation.

Method: First, make a cup of ginger tea with water, sliced ginger, honey, and lemon or lime juice. Then mixture 1 tbsp. Of castor oil within the tea and drink each night time time time in advance than mattress for three days.

Chapter 17: image-placeholder

Autophagy way self-eating It is coined from automobile (regarding self) and phagy (eating/devouring). Autophagy may be defined as how our frame reshapes and rebuilds itself, removing unwanted additives. The technique of autophagy includes the body breaking down and destroying vintage, damaged, and diseased cells and then recycling that cellular fabric into new, healthy cells.

Autophagy is a device your frame uses to interrupt down pollutants. This is your body's recycling system. Once pollution building up, they cause various sicknesses. Autophagy permits you avoid those ailments with the useful resource of cleansing your device.

The technique is form of constant and tremendously extended while we're younger, however as we begin to age, autophagy simply slows down. This slowing down of the autophagy technique basically outcomes in developing older in people, and the collect of diseased and broken cells contributes to diseases which incorporates most cancers,

Alzheimer's, and fantastic degenerative illnesses.

Recent research have found out a hyperlink among fasting and autophagy. Autophagy takes vicinity in all cells within the body. When we speedy, in preference to digesting meals, our body focuses on outlining the pollutants and cellular count that are not beneficial to our fitness. This cleaning way will start with the most realty obtained or superior poisons after which move directly to the older pollutants. So the longer you may rapid, the more headway can be made in detoxifying your frame.

Autophagy is the frame's manner of cleansing itself out. The system consists of small "hunter" particles that circulate spherical your body seeking out cells or cell additives which might be vintage and broken. The hunter particles then take these cell additives aside, disposing of the broken factors and saving the precious quantities to make new cells later. These hunter cells also can use beneficial leftover abilities to create strength for the frame.

The one-of-a-kind characteristic that autophagy serves is that it lets in cells carry out their loss of life at the same time as it is time to die. There are times at the equal time as cells are programmed to die due to numerous various factors. Sometimes those cells need assist in their lack of life, and autophagy can help them with this or can help to easy up after their death. The human body is all about lifestyles and loss of life, and those strategies are continuously taking region without our knowledge to preserve us healthful and in suitable shape.

Types of autophagy

There are three significant types of autophagy: macro-autophagy, micro-autophagy, and chaperone autophagy.

•Macro-autophagy: Its sports are completed in masses of cell components. Macro-autophagy is split into : bulk and selective.

•Micro-autophagy: It is more specialized. It includes the direct engulfment of decided on substances. This may be foreign places bodies which includes substances, bacteria, or any element alien to the body.

•Chaperone autophagy: This is the most complex form of autophagy. For chaperone autophagy to occur, a specific protein known as hsc70 want to be present.

Intermittent fasting triggers autophagy

Autophagy generally starts offevolved after a 24-hour fast, after your frame has used up all the gas needed to rejuvenate and rebuild cells. This also can variety for special people, relying on the carbohydrate tiers of your healthy eating plan earlier than the quick and exercising ordinary. Once your body reaches this aspect, autophagy starts offevolved offevolved offevolved to arise. This device is evolutionary and adapting in nature, in which your frame will first select out damaged cells, tissues, pollution, and similar materials to break down first.

These items are then recycled and rebuilt into new, stronger cells in their place. The new cells are greater efficient and greater more youthful, in which the anti-growing older benefit takes impact. Healthier, extra immature cells construct higher tissues to your body's organs, enhancing function and normal appearance as a give up give up end result.

The health advantages of autophagy

1. The removal of pollutants from cells, breaking down damaged cells, and reusing or recycling them have the impact of stopping Alzheimer's and Parkinson's sickness, which is probably attributed to poisonous protein assemble-up in cells. Breaking the ones proteins down is essential to prevention.

2. Another advantage of breaking down damaged cells may additionally additionally prevent or perhaps address some styles of maximum cancers. Studies show that retaining healthful, vital cells can play a giant role in lowering the risk of most cancers. During autophagy, the damaged cells are the number one materials to be damaged down, casting off the opportunities of developing and multiplying. In effect, cancerous cells are removed and destroyed through autophagy.

three. It is the very last detox and cleansing approach. Autophagy detoxes the frame at a cellular diploma, that is a long way greater powerful in project consequences.

four. Autophagy slows down the developing older approach. By rejuvenating cells on a extra green and common basis through ordinary fasting cycles, your pores and pores and pores and skin will become clearer, your thoughts more centered, and your frame more younger.

image-placeholder

Benefits of intermittent fasting

•Weight loss: When you rapid, your frame's insulin production lowers and motives your body cells to launch their glucose shops as strength. So if you fast often, you'll keep to shed pounds.

•Lowers your threat of diabetes: Fasting permits you shed pounds and influences various factors that boom your hazard of kind 2 diabetes. Studies display that intermittent fasting help decrease every blood glucose and insulin degrees in diabetes patients and overweight humans.

•Lowers oxidative strain and contamination in the body: Oxidative pressure can cause untimely developing vintage and diverse chronic illnesses, however intermittent fasting can decrease oxidative strain and help lower contamination. It is the contamination that triggers all forms of modern-day situations.

•Improves coronary coronary coronary heart health: Researchers placed that intermittent fasting have to motive a discount in triglycerides, ldl ldl ldl cholesterol, coronary coronary heart price, and blood strain.

•Improved thoughts fitness: Animal studies show that intermittent fasting improves thoughts health and reminiscence. Other studies show that fasting can suppress inflammation within the mind. The contamination motives neurological conditions which includes Alzheimer's disease, Parkinson's ailment, and stroke. Studies show that fasting can lower the threat of these illnesses.

•Fasting induces numerous mobile repair strategies: When we rapid, our our our bodies provoke a way known as autophagy. During autophagy, the frame eliminates waste and poisonous substances. Repeated autophagy can defend our frame closer to numerous illnesses, along with Alzheimer's and maximum cancers.

•Lowers your risk of most cancers: Animal studies display that fasting can lessen most cancers risk. Also, human studies display that intermittent fasting can decrease the facet results of chemotherapy.

Fasted country

When the human body is in a fasted u . S ., it has numerous strategies to offer strength. Glucose is the body's default gas, which comes from carb and sugar-rich elements and is saved as glycogen. Liver glycogen stores are depleted in the first 18 to 24 hours of fasting. This extensively decreases blood sugar and insulin degrees.

George Cahill, a primary expert in fasting frame form, describes this approach more virtually:

•Feeding: We devour carb-wealthy food; they convert to glucose inside the frame. Our blood sugar/glucose levels bypass up, and insulin degrees upward push to transport glucose into cells. Additional glucose is stored as glycogen inside the liver or saved as body fats.

•The submit-absorptive segment: Usually, this kingdom is activated 4 hours after a meal. Both blood sugar and insulin tiers begin to fall. Consequently, the liver breaks down glycogen to deliver power to the body.

•Gluconeogenesis: sixteen hours into the short. At this element, glycogen shops start to lessen. Glucose levels fall but stay inside the ordinary variety.

•Ketosis: The frame's glucose tiers lessen, and the liver starts offevolved offevolved to break down frame-fat storage into fatty acids, then breaks down the ones fatty acids into an power-wealthy detail known as ketones or ketone our our bodies. The presence of ketone our bodies within the blood is called ketosis.

20, 24 hours, and 36 hours fast

The Warrior Diet or 20-hour speedy:

Ori Hofmekler is the inventor of this fasting protocol. He is an professional on survival technology and a supporter of intermittent fasting. With this protocol, you rapid for about 20 hours each day and then devour a massive meal at night time. The Warrior Diet shadows the Paleolithic life-style of our ancestors. During the 20-hour fast, you can consume a few portions of raw fruit or greens. You also can consume a few servings of protein if preferred.

Eat Stop Eat or 24-hour speedy:

Brad Pilon invented this fasting protocol. He is a fasting enthusiast and one of the worldwide's main supporters of intermittent fasting. With this method, you fast for an entire of 24 hours some times every week. The inventor Brad Pilon refers to this system as a "24 ruin from ingesting". Once your speedy is over, you can start to consume typically. Some want to devour a moderate snack after the fast; others want to interrupt the short with a big meal.

36-hour fast:

This speedy is also referred to as Monk fast. It is finished once consistent with week. More than weight reduction, this rapid targets to get a clearer thoughts and a lift in cognitive function. A 36-hour rapid gives you extraordinary weight loss benefits. After sixteen hours of fasting, the human frame breaks down body fats for strength. You get the maximum fat-burning blessings among sixteen and 28 hours of fasting.

image-placeholder

Ayurvedic speedy

1. Choosing the tremendous time: If you awaken in the morning and study any sort of digestive problems which includes burning, bloating, burping, or gas, you may start a quick to treatment it. Fasting will deliver your digestive gadget a rest and permit your frame to take away ama.

2. The doshas: Ayurveda approves brief, everyday fasting. Ayurveda discourages prolonged durations of fasting due to the reality it may create a disconnect among your mind and frame. It also can cause health troubles that might take months to heal. Ayurveda recommends a fruit or juice speedy for maximum people. It says that absolute fasting isn't always for anyone.

three. Fasting for Vata: Fasting can provoke Vata through developing mild, dry and bloodless developments. Avoid water fasting or fasting for two days when you have a Vata imbalance. According to Ayurveda, you need to fast as soon as a month. Eat mango, candy orange, or grape juice all through your fast – all of them are Vata pacifying.

four. Fasting for Pitta: Choose a juice speedy of bitter and astringent vegetables. Drink pomegranate, grape, prune juice, or juices made from leafy greens. Do in the future fast every week and a three day fast at the alternate of the seasons.

five. Fasting for Kapha: If you are in right health, then you can practice three-day fasttimes a 3 hundred and sixty five days. Drink warm water, lemon-honey drink, or apple and cranberry juice during your fast. You can practice a 1-day speedy as soon as every week.

General guidelines for achievement

•If you feel indignant, depleted, inclined, or painfully hungry at some point of your fast, then harm your speedy.

•Eat your largest meal at lunchtime, even even as you're fasting.

•Eat simplest at the same time as you are hungry

•Drink tea crafted from coriander, cumin, and fennel seeds. This tea ignites your digestive fireside and lets in put off pollutants.

•Consume Triphala all through your rapid. Triphala helps the digestive device, acts as a moderate detoxifier, and promotes healthful elimination

•Ideally, you need to pick out out the same day for fasting each week.

•During your fast, you could experience moderate-headed or a touch tired. These are commonplace signs and signs and could leave on their very own. If the ones signs and symptoms come to be immoderate, then spoil your rapid.

•Take more relaxation in some unspecified time in the future of your fast. Practice meditation and journaling

How to cease your fast

Do not consume your normal meals while you smash your fast. Eat a fruit or a small amount of warm cereal if breakfast time. Then consume a clean lunch in the path of lunchtime. For instance, in case you plan to speedy for 2 days, then consume a lighter, cleanser weight loss program earlier than and after your fast.

Who need to now not speedy?

•Children

•Very aged

•Pregnant

- Breastfeeding

- Menstruating

- Underweight or undernourished

- Have a continual contamination

image-placeholder

Glowing Ageless Skin

Typical factors for pores and pores and pores and skin issues:

- Repressed feelings

- Anxiety, worry, fear

- Anger, contamination, frustration

- Lowered immunity

- Lack of sleep

- High stress

- Alcohol or drug use

- Using harsh face wash or cleansing cleansing cleaning soap

- External irritants together with chemical compounds, detergents, or perfumes

- Eating allergic components

- Excessive warmth in the blood or liver

- Toxins within the blood or liver

- Toxins within the device

- Digestion problems

- Liver troubles

- Negativity

Dietary hints for wholesome pores and pores and pores and skin

1. Avoid allergenic, aggravating substances: Some common culprits are nuts, eggs, components, preservatives, gluten, wheat, sugar, soy, and dairy.

2. Eat hydrating, cooling ingredients: You need to devour cooling meals to help stability out the extra warmth within the gadget. Consume hydrating, cooling materials which include pomegranate, watermelon, parsley, cilantro, lime, natural ghee, coconut oil, and bitter vegetables collectively with collards, chard, and kale.

3. Avoid heating materials: Avoid heating acidic or quite spiced materials. Some examples encompass citrus fruit (besides lime), peppers, nightshades (eggplant, potato, tomato), fried meals, alcohol, fermented meals, vinegar, and notably salty substances. Avoid spices which includes ajwain, cayenne pepper, fenugreek, cinnamon, dry ginger, and black pepper.

4. Lime water: Drink 16 ouncesWarm lime water inside the morning. This drink will increase digestion, detoxifies the body and balances Pitta.

five. Eat antioxidant-wealthy meals: Eat colorful quit result and vegetables each day. Some of the incredible options are pomegranate, blueberries, strawberries, cucumber, sprouts, bitter vegetables, pumpkin, candy potato, beets, summer season squash, glowing turmeric, and smooth ginger.

6. Avoid unsuitable food combos: This is one of the number one reasons of sicknesses. Wrong food combos reason poisonous construct-up and purpose infections.

Lifestyle pointers for healthful pores and skin

1. Ayurveda oil rubdown: Perform Ayurveda oil rubdown or Abhyanga each night time time earlier than bed. If you're experiencing itchiness, dryness, eczema, or stupid pores and skin, then use Pitta massage oil or coconut oil to rubdown the affected regions in advance than mattress every night time.

2. Steam tub: Taking a steam bathtub or sauna more than one instances every week is a extraordinary way to increase pass, remove pollutants and hydrate the pores and skin.

three. Exercise: Exercise 3 instances every week (30 minutes each time). Regular workout will boom circulate, and it's miles a herbal manner to detoxify the frame. Walk unexpectedly or use a treadmill.

4. Yoga: Practicing yoga is a wonderful manner to increase drift and detoxify the frame. Start your day with 15 to 20 minutes of mild yoga exercise.

five. Meditate: Daily meditation offers many health advantages, which includes glowing pores and pores and skin. Practice meditation for 10 to fifteen minutes every morning.

6. Avoid direct sun publicity: Direct sun exposure can harm your pores and skin. If you need to skip outdoor, use sunscreen, placed on a hat, and proper apparel.

Herbal treatments for healthy pores and skin

1. Tikta Ghrita: This is likewise called sour ghee. This ghee is used to enhance the complexion and heal the pores and pores and skin. In ½ cup heat water, mixture ½ tsp. Of this ghee and drink on an empty belly each morning.

2. Triphala Churna: This natural remedy improves pores and skin situations. Mix ½ tsp. Of this components in a ½ cup of warmth water and drink every night time time time in advance than mattress. You can also make a paste with Triphala Churna and apply it to your face to increase the pores and skin's radiance.

3. Aloe vera juice: You can drink this juice or workout it right away on your pores and pores and pores and skin. Take 1 tbsp. Of

herbal aloe vera gel 3 instances every day earlier than meals for 1 month. You can add a pinch of neem and turmeric for even extra remarkable results.

4. Cooling herbs for wholesome, radiant, clean pores and skin:

•Tikta

•Karalla

•Aloe

•Shankhpushpi

•Bhringaraj

•Bhumyamalaki

•Amalaki

•Kalmegh

•Turmeric

•Neem

•Kutiki

five. Detoxifying herbs:

•Shilajit

- Vidanga

- Triphala Guggulu

- Neem

- Manjistha

- Guduchi

- Musta

6. Digestive herbs: Robust digestive fitness is essential for radiant pores and pores and pores and skin

- Turmeric

- Cardamom

- Coriander

- Fennel

- Pippali

- Ginger

- Chitrak

7. Antioxidant-wealthy herbs enhance pores and pores and skin fitness;

- Elderberry

- Rosemary

- Clove

- Daruharidra

- Ginger

- Shilajit

- Turmeric

- Hibiscus

- Rose Hips

- Amalaki

Improving your pores and skin fitness

1. Eat a balanced weight loss program and on time. Eating a balanced food plan will assist your liver and kidneys detoxify your frame.

2. Drink carrot juice: Carrots are wealthy in vitamins and antioxidants and help decorate the fitness of your pores and pores and skin. Drink a tumbler of carrot juicetimes every day on an empty belly for 15 to twenty days.

3. Neem: Mix 1 tsp. Neem powder in a cup of warmth water and drink two times every day on an empty stomach.

4. Manjistha Powder: This herb permits the liver detoxify the body and enhance pores and skin state of affairs. Mix 1 tsp. Manjistha powder in a cup of warm water and drink 2 instances every day on an empty stomach.

five. Fasting: Fasting can decorate your pores and pores and skin scenario. Try to rapid as quickly as in step with week.

6. Guduchi: This herb additionally facilitates beautify your pores and skin health. If you are taking this herb's pill shape, take 1 pill 2 times a day on an empty belly. If you are taking the powder shape, devour it with warm water half-hour after your food.

image-placeholder

An Ayurvedic approach to healthful hair

Here are the motives for terrible hair health and hair loss;

•Prescription tablets

•Hypothyroidism

•Poor circulate

•Iron deficiency anemia

- Excessive pollutants inside the device

- Poor liver health

- Poor digestion

- Doshic imbalance

- Hormonal imbalance

- Lack of sleep

- Stress

- Genetics

An Ayurvedic healthy eating plan for wholesome hair

1. Boost digestion: Brittle hair and hair loss are frequently because of excessive ama (pollutants) in the system. You need to enhance your digestion electricity to growth the absorption of essential vitamins and burn off pollutants.

2. Bone nourishing minerals and vitamins: Eat a diet plan rich in bone nourishing nutrients and minerals. According to Ayurveda, hair is the spinoff of the bones. Some vital vitamins and minerals to embody on your weight-reduction plan are boron, magnesium, zinc,

potassium, calcium, Vitamin B, Vitamin C, Vitamin D, and Vitamin K. Try no longer to take nutritional nutritional supplements. Omega – three fatty acids are also critical.

3. Consume healthful oils: Healthy oils will nourish your hair from the internal out. The great oils are sesame oil, olive oil, almond oil, coconut oil, and ghee.

4. Include wholesome dairy: They embody hair-satisfactory proteins, Vitamin B5 and Vitamin D.

5. Eat nuts and seeds every day: Eating nuts and seeds will enhance your hair health. The great nuts and seeds are almonds, walnuts, sunflower seeds, pumpkin seeds, and sesame seeds.

6. Eat colourful end result and greens every day: Try to devour a rainbow of healthful culmination and vegetables. They provide nutrients, minerals, and antioxidants critical for hair health. Some awesome alternatives are bitter vegetables, cucumbers, carrots, crimson cauliflower, red potatoes, bell peppers, sweet potatoes, melon,

strawberries, blueberries, mangoes, ripe bananas, dates, coconut, and soaked raisins.

7. Add spices in your meals: Some hair-healthy alternatives are cloves, nutmeg, cardamom, cinnamon, mustard seed, fenugreek, ajwain, cumin, pippali, black pepper, ginger, turmeric, and Agni Churna.

8. Stay hydrated: This is crucial for healthy hair growth. Drink 6 to eight/ cups of natural, heat water every day. Avoid cold and iced liquids. Instead, drink coconut water, herbal teas, and cucumber juice.

An Ayurvedic manner of existence for healthy hair

1. Manage strain: Lowering strain can enhance hair fitness. Practice deep breathing bodily sports, meditation, and yoga. Also, surrounding yourself with cherished ones and on foot in nature lets in.

2. Scalp massage: Massage your scalp with warmth oil each night time in advance than mattress. This will boom hair health. Use Sunflower oil for Kapha, sesame oil for Vata, and coconut oil for Pitta.

three. Regular bowel actions: Drink loads of water and fiber-wealthy components to take away constipation. Regular bowel movements are essential for hair fitness.

four. Avoid immoderate sun publicity: Excessive sun publicity increases the Pitta in the frame and results in hair loss. Avoid immoderate sun publicity.

five. Brush your hair: Brush your hair severa times every day. This will growth the growth and fitness of your hair.

Ayurvedic herbs for healthy hair

• Bhringaraj

• Amalaki

• Guduchi

• Yesti Madhura

• Brahmi

• Bala

• Ashwagandha

The reasons for hair loss;

• Over styling

- Poor food plan

- Excessive strain

- Lifestyle and environmental elements

- Genetics

- Age

- Hormones

Ayurvedic techniques to make your hair increase longer

1. First, decide your dosha imbalances. This will help you already know what's causing your hair troubles.

2. Condition your hair with Kesha Dravyas in advance than hair wash: Kesha Dravyas includes the subsequent materials. These factors enhance hair fitness:

- Amala

- Brahmi

- Jatamansi

- Neelini

- Bhringraj

•Sesame seeds

•Coconut

Massage your scalp and hair with herbal oils crafted from the above elements. Then wash your hair. You also can exercise eggs, aloe vera gel, yogurt, and henna paste on your scalp and hair. Then wash it after a while.

three. Use Ayurvedic or herbal shampoo: Use an Ayurvedic shampoo that consists of the subsequent elements:

•Shikakai (cleansing cleaning soap pod): Shikakai gets rid of more oil and pollutants from your scalp. You can use Shikakai with Reetha (cleaning soap nut) and Amla.

•Hibiscus leaves and plants: The hibiscus leaves and flower paste gather properly-nourished, lengthy hair.

•Aloe vera: Aloe vera allows easy the scalp and may be very useful in treating imbalance.

•Triphala Churna: The blend of Shikakai (soap pod), Reetha (cleaning soap nut), and Triphala churna is a number of the first rate herbal shampoos for the hair.

four. Professional Ayurvedic remedy plans:

Takradhara: This Ayurvedic method stops hair fall and untimely greying. You pour a go with the flow of medicated buttermilk over the forehead with this manner.

Basti: This approach makes use of medicated herbal oils to pacify Vata dosha inside the colon and decorate hair health.

5. At-domestic Ayurvedic treatments:

•Nasya: This tool consists of setting natural oil drops in the nostril. Nasya permits to detox your head and upkeep broken hair.

•Pichu: In this approach, you soak a cotton gauze pad with warmness Ayurvedic oil and comply with it over your Crown chakra.

•Karnabhyanga: This method consists of ear massage with oil. This rub down calms your mind and allows fight hair fall because of Vata.

•Padabhyanga: This technique includes massaging your toes with herbal oil. This rubdown lowers more Pitta dosha and stops hair fall. You can also carry out Kansa Vatki for your feet. With this method, you use a steel bowl crafted from tin, zinc, and copper to rub onto and simulate your ft. This can also beautify hair health.

•Scalp scrubbing: This manner removes pollutants out of your scalp and promotes blood motion and hair boom. Some of the elements you can use for scalp scrubbing:

•A mixture of sugar and honey

•Fenugreek powder

•A mixture of onion and honey

•A blend of freshly chopped ginger and black pepper

www.ingramcontent.com/pod-product-compliance
Lightning Source LLC
Chambersburg PA
CBHW060500030426
42337CB00015B/1664